柔道整復師のための英会話表現

塩川春彦 執筆代表／杉山　渉・小黒正幸 監修

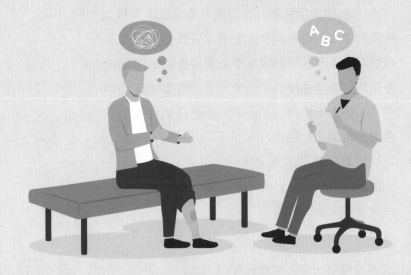

本日はどうされましたか.
What brings you here today?

この範囲を固定していきます.
I will immobilize this area.

患部を動かさないようにしてください.
You must try not to move the injured part.

医歯薬出版株式会社

執筆代表

塩川　春彦　元 帝京科学大学医療科学部東京柔道整復学科 教授

監　修

杉山　渉　帝京科学大学医療科学部東京柔道整復学科 教授
小黒　正幸　帝京科学大学医療科学部東京柔道整復学科 講師

執筆者一覧

有賀　雅史　帝京科学大学医療科学部東京柔道整復学科 教授
市毛　雅之　帝京科学大学医療科学部柔道整復学科 教授
二神　弘子　帝京科学大学医療科学部東京柔道整復学科 教授
大石　徹　防衛大学校総合教育学群体育学教育室 准教授
行田　直人　帝京科学大学医療科学部東京柔道整復学科 准教授
登本　茂芳　元 帝京科学大学医療科学部東京柔道整復学科 准教授
濱田　淳　帝京科学大学医療科学部東京柔道整復学科 准教授
畑山　元政　帝京科学大学医療科学部東京柔道整復学科 講師
佐藤　勉　帝京科学大学医療科学部東京柔道整復学科 講師
浅木　健治　帝京科学大学医療科学部東京柔道整復学科 助教
原　朋弘　帝京千住接骨院院長
高嶋　洋友　AHT＆R高嶋 代表兼フリーランス・トレーナー
黒坂竜乃介　三鷹整形外科リハビリテーション科
五十嵐大真　帝京千住大橋接骨院

英文校閲

Antonija Cavcic　滋賀県立大学人間文化学部 講師

This book is originally published in Japanese
under the title of :

JUDOSEIFUKUSHINOTAMENO EIKAIWAHYOGEN

(English Conversation for Judo Therapists)

SHIOKAWA, Haruhiko
Former Professor, Teikyo University of Science

© 2022 1st ed.
ISHIYAKU PUBLISHERS, INC.
  7-10, Honkomagome 1 chome, Bunkyo-ku,
  Tokyo 113-8612, Japan

序

　日本に居住する外国人の数が増え，外国人の患者が接骨院を訪れる機会も増加しています．

　本書は，柔道整復師が日本語を話すことができない外国人患者に対して柔道整復術を行えるよう，接骨院でのコミュニケーションに必要な英語表現を収集したものです．読者対象は，専門学校や大学で柔道整復術を学ぶ学生，および現役の柔道整復師の皆さんです．

　在日外国人の誰もが英語を母語としているわけではありませんが，英語を第二言語として話す外国人はたくさんいます．ですから，柔道整復師が患者とのコミュニケーションを図るための英語表現を学ぶことは十分な意義があります．

　本書では，外国人患者とのコミュニケーションに必要な英語表現について，できるだけ多くの例文を収録することを心掛けました．本書を利用する皆さんには，じっくりと時間をかけてさまざまな英語表現を学んでほしいと願っています．より多くの英語表現を知っていれば，患者への説明がより詳細なものになり，一方，患者の訴えをより正確に理解できるようになります．このことは，より円滑な施術へとつながります．また，現役の柔道整復師のなかには，仕事上必要な英語表現をもっと学びたいと思う方々もいらっしゃるでしょう．本書は，そのような方がたにも役立つものです．

　本書を使って学ぶことにより，優れた英語コミュニケーション力も備えた柔道整復師が増えることを期待します．

　なお，内容の正確性，適切性を保持するためにできる限りの努力をしましたが，修正すべき箇所や改善すべき箇所があるかもしれません．読者のみなさまからのフィードバックをいただければ幸いです．

2022年9月

著　者

本書作成の経緯

　本書作成の過程は，以下のとおりです．

　本書の執筆代表である塩川は，帝京科学大学医療科学部東京柔道整復学科の必修科目「基礎医療英語」を，学科開設年の2010年より担当し，柔道整復術を学ぶ学生が将来の職業生活上必要と思われる英語を授業で扱うべく，英語教材を作ってきました．その過程において，東京柔道整復学科に所属する教員，および附属接骨院に所属する柔道整復師に協力を仰ぎ，接骨院でよく使われる日本語表現例の充実と整理を図りました．収集された日本語表現は塩川によって英訳され，それに対し本書作成に参加した教員陣からフィードバックが与えられ，改訂が重ねられました．その間，本書監修者の杉山，小黒によって内容の正確性と適切性を高める努力が続けられ，本書の完成に至りました．

著　者

柔道整復について説明するための表現
Expressions to Describe Judo Therapy

Introduction

接骨院を訪れる外国人は，柔道整復施術について熟知していない可能性があります．接骨院での英会話表現を学ぶ前に，序章として柔道整復施術の概要，特徴を説明する英語表現を紹介します．柔道整復師として自分の仕事の概要を外国人に英語で説明したい場面は，国際化した社会では必ずあります．柔道整復師は医師ではないので麻酔（anesthesia）や注射（injection）を使えず，施術はnon-invasive（非観血的）なものである，というようなことを英語で伝えられるようにしておきましょう．

柔道整復とは

柔道整復は，骨折，脱臼，打撲，および捻挫などを治療する方法のひとつです．

Judo therapy is one of the methods of treating broken or dislocated bones, contusions, sprains, and so on.

> therapy：施術，療法 / method：方法 / broken (bone)：折れた（骨）/ dislocated bone：脱臼した骨 / contusion：打撲 / sprain：捻挫（→ p35, One Point「主な傷病・症状」）

柔道整復は，世界保健機関（WHO）の報告書＊で日本の伝統的な医療のひとつとして言及されています．

Judo therapy is cited as one of Japan's traditional medical treatments in a report* from the World Health Organization (WHO).

> cite：言及する / traditional medicine：伝統医療 / organization：機関，組織

*Legal Status of Traditional Medicine and Complementary/Alternative Medicine: A Worldwide Review (WHO, 2001)『伝統医療と相補・代替医療に関する報告』（世界保健機関，2001年）

柔道整復は柔道にその起源をもちますが，近現代以降，東洋医学よりも現代の西洋医学の一部として発展してきました．

Judo therapy has its origins in judo, but since the modern era, it has developed as a part of modern western medicine rather than oriental medicine.

> origin：起源 / the modern era：近現代 / develop：発展する / western medicine：西洋医学

柔道整復の施術では，施術者は薬の使用，麻酔，注射，エックス線の使用ができず，また手術ができません．

In judo therapy treatments, therapists are not allowed to use medicines, anesthesia, injections, X-rays, or perform surgery.

> therapist：施術者 / allow：許す / medicine：薬 / anesthesia：麻酔 / injection：注射 / surgery：手術 / X-ray：エックス線

柔道整復の施術は非観血的なものです．

Judo therapy treatments are non-invasive.

> non-invasive：非観血的（血を見ることのない），手術をしない ↔ invasive：観血的，手術をする

柔道整復師は，状態を注意深く確かめ，患部に直接触れることで患者を施術します．

Judo therapists treat patients by carefully checking the patient's condition and directly touching the affected area.

> patient：患者 / directly：直接に / affected area：患部

≡ 柔道整復師とは

医師と，専門教育を受けた柔道整復師だけが柔道整復を行うことができます．

Only medical doctors and professionally-trained judo therapists can practice judo therapy.

> professionally-trained：専門教育（専門的訓練）を受けた / practice：実践する

柔道整復師は厚生労働省によって公認された職業です．

Judo therapy is an occupation* certified by the Ministry of Health, Labor and Welfare.

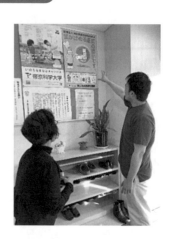

> occupation：職業 / certify：公認する / the Ministry of Health, Labor and Welfare：厚生労働省

＊occupation（＝職業）は，人をさす言葉ではなく，仕事の内容をさす言葉なので，この文では主語に judo therapy を用いる．

国家試験に合格した者だけが，柔道整復の施術を行うことができます．

Only those who have passed the national exam can perform judo therapy treatments.

> those who ～：～である人々 / national exam：国家試験 / perform = practice：行う

柔道整復師養成学校には大学および専門学校があり，大学では4年間の，専門学校では3年間の教育課程があります．そこでは，柔道整復に必要な特別な技能の他に，解剖学，生理学，病理学，衛生学などを教えます．

Training schools of judo therapy include universities and vocational schools: universities have four-year programs, and vocational schools have three-year programs. Those schools teach anatomy, physiology, pathology, hygiene, and so on, in addition to special skills necessary for judo therapy.

> anatomy：解剖学 / physiology：生理学 / pathology：病理学 / hygiene：衛生学 / special skills necessary for 〜：〜にとって必要な特別な技能

柔道整復を実践する者のほとんどは，接骨院と呼ばれる施術施設で働いています．

Most practitioners of judo therapy work for a treatment facility called *sekkotsu-in*.

> practitioner：実践者 / treatment facility：施術施設

一部の柔道整復師は，病院などの医療機関で働いています．柔道整復師は，介護施設，スポーツジム，プロスポーツなどでも活躍しています．

Some judo therapists work for medical institutions, such as hospitals. Judo therapists also work for care facilities, sports gyms, and in the professional sports industry.

> medical institution：医療機関

1 受付のための表現
Expressions for Registration

受付は，接骨院を訪れる人とコミュニケーションをとるスタートですから，とても大切です．ここで外国人の患者を困惑させたり，不安にさせたりしてはいけません．受付では，施術申込書（registration form）への記入のお願い，緊急の場合の連絡（contact 〜 in case of an emergency），保険証（health insurance card）についての説明，医療措置でない施術（non-medical treatment）の説明など，誤解のないように伝えなければならないことがいくつもあります．

受付

おはようございます．/ こんにちは．/ こんばんは．
Good morning. / Good afternoon. / Good evening.

はじめての来院ですか．/ こちらに来院されたことがありますか．
Is this your first visit here? / Have you ever been here before?

visit：訪問 → 来院

再来院ですか．
Is this your return visit?

return visit：再診

いつ来院されましたか．/ 前回の来院はいつでしたか．/
こちらに前回いらしたのはいつですか．
**When did you visit us? / When was the last time you came here? /
When was it that you came here last?**

再来院の方は施術券を出してください．
If this is not your first visit [If this is a return visit], please show me your patient ID card.

patient ID card：診察券 → 施術券

他の医療機関からの紹介状をお持ちですか.

Do you have a referral from another medical facility?

referral：紹介状

One
Point

靴に関する表現

靴を脱いでください.　Please take off your shoes.
靴は靴箱に入れてください.　Please put your shoes in the shoebox.
靴はそこに置いてください.　Please put your shoes over there.
スリッパを履いてください.　Please put on the slippers.

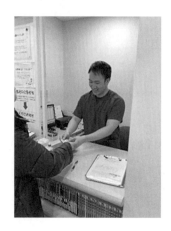

施術申込書

こちらが記入していただく施術申込書になります.

Here is a registration form for you to fill out.

registration form：施術申込書（→p94, 巻末付録（5））/ fill out：記入する

（この）施術申込書に記入してください.

Please fill out the [this] registration form.

施術申込書を確認させていただきます.

Let me check your registration form.

施術申込書の一番上の欄に住所を記入してください.

Please fill in your home address at the top of the form.

あなたの名前と住所を記入してください.

Could you write your name and home address, please?

施術申込書の一番下に勤務先の電話番号を記入してください.

Please fill in your office phone number at the bottom.

ここにあなたのフルネームをご記入ください.

Please write down your first name, middle name, and last name here. /
I need you to write your name in full.

Jamie というのは名字ですか.

Is Jamie your family name?

どちらが名字ですか.

Which of these is your last name?

この電話番号で昼間に連絡が取れますか.

Can I reach you at this number during the daytime?

> reach 〜：〜に連絡をとる

日中に連絡が取れる電話番号を教えてください.

What is your daytime telephone number?

携帯電話の番号を教えてください.

Can you tell me your cellular phone number?

> cellular phone：携帯電話

緊急の場合はどなたに連絡を取ればいいですか.

Whom may I contact in case of an emergency?

> contact：連絡をとる / in case of an emergency：緊急の場合に

緊急時には会社にご連絡してもよろしいですか.

In case of an emergency, can I make a phone call to your company?

健康保険証

（日本の）健康保険に加入していますか．
Do you have (Japanese national) health insurance?
`health insurance：健康保険`

保険の証書を見せていただけますか．
May I see proof of your insurance?
`proof：証書`

健康保険証をお持ちになられていますか．
Do you have your health insurance card with you?
`health insurance card：健康保険証`

健康保険証を見せてください．/ 受付の者に保険証を見せてください．
Please show me your health insurance card. /
You have to show your insurance card to the clerk.
`clerk：事務員`

申込書と健康保険証を受付に出してください．
Please hand in your application form and health insurance card to the reception desk.
`application form：申込書 / reception desk：受付`

保険に加入されていないので，全額をご負担いただきます．
Since you don't have any health insurance, we will ask that you pay the full fee.
`ask that 〜：〜であることを要求する / full fee：全額`

次回は保険証を必ず持ってきてください．
Don't forget to bring your health insurance card next time.
`forget to 〜：〜することを忘れる`

外国人登録がお済みで，かつ日本に 1 年以上居住されるご予定でしたら，国民健康保険と国民年金に登録申請をすることができます．

If you have registered as a foreign-resident and plan to live in Japan for longer than a year, you can apply to enroll into the National Health Insurance program and the National Pension program.

register as a foreign-resident：外国人登録を済ませる / apply to enroll into 〜：〜への登録申請をする / the National Health Insurance program：国民健康保険 / the National Pension program：国民年金

医療措置ではない施術は健康保険が適用されません．医療措置ではない施術には，肩こり，疲労による腰痛を緩和すること，慰安のためのマッサージなどが含まれます．

Non-medical treatments are not covered by health insurance. Those non-medical treatments include treatments to ease stiff shoulders and back pain caused by fatigue, massage to ease stress, and so on.

non-medical treatment：医療措置でない施術 / ease：緩和する / stiff shoulders：肩こり（→p35, One Point「主な傷病・症状」）/ back pain caused by fatigue：疲労による腰痛 / massage：マッサージ / ease stress：ストレスを癒す

質問票への記入

こちらの質問票に記入してください．

Please fill in the medical questionnaire [patient consultation sheet].

medical questionnaire ＝ patient consultation sheet：質問票（→p92-93，巻末付録（4））

（名前が）呼ばれるまでこちらでお待ちください．

Please wait here until you are called [until your name is called].

2 医療面接のための表現
Expressions for Medical consultations

Introduction

医療面接は，適切な施術をするための判断材料を得るものです．患者の主訴（chief complaint）を理解するための適切な質問表現，患者の主訴にありがちな英語表現をあらかじめ知っておくべきでしょう．また，捻挫する（sprain），〜を打撲する（have a bruise on 〜）など，けがの描写の表現，「膝を曲げると痛む」（When I bend my knee, it hurts），「ギクッとする（激しく痛む）」（have a sharp pain）のような痛みを描写する頻出表現を覚えましょう．

≡ 医療面接の開始

施術室へお入りください．
Please enter the treatment room.

> treatment room：施術室

本日施術を担当いたします小林と申します．
My name is [I am] Kobayashi, I will be in charge of your treatment today.

> be in charge of 〜：〜を担当する

こちらにおかけください．
Please take a seat here.

本日はどうされましたか．
What brings you here today? / What can I do for you today? / How can I help you today?

なにが問題でしょうか．
Have you had any problems? / What seems to be the trouble?

患者の主訴を理解する

左足首を捻挫したようです.
I think I have sprained my left ankle.

足をひねったのですが, ちょっと診ていただけますか.
I twisted my foot, and I would like to see if it's all right.

> twist：ひねる / see if it is all right：大丈夫かどうか診る

つまずいて, 打ち身をつくってしまいました.
I stumbled and bruised myself.

> stumble：つまずく / bruise：打撲する（→ p35, One Point「主な傷病・症状」）

30分ぐらい前に階段から転げ落ちた時, 肩の骨を外したようです.
When I fell down the steps about 30 minutes ago, I felt as if I had dislocated my shoulder.

> fall down the steps：階段から転げ落ちる / dislocate：脱臼する

寝ちがえて, 首が回りません.
I got a crick in my neck while sleeping.

> get a crick in one's neck：首が痛くなる

*痛みに焦点を絞った表現は, p15を参照.

けがに焦点を絞った表現

どこをけがしましたか（痛めましたか）.
Where are you hurt? / Where are you injured?

> be hurt：痛める / be injured：けがをする

どのようにしてけがをしましたか（痛めましたか）.
How did the injury occur?

> occur：起きる

それはいつ起きましたか.
When did it happen?

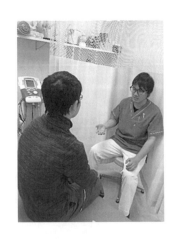

なにか原因はありますか.

Was there any cause?

> cause：原因, 引き起こす

なんらかの無理をしたのではありませんか.

Have you strained yourself in any way?

> strain oneself：無理をする / in any way：なんらかの方法で

最近激しいスポーツに参加していませんか.

Have you been participating in vigorous sports recently?

> participate：参加する / vigorous：活気あふれる / recently：最近

→週末にゴルフをやりますが, それだけです.

On the weekends I play golf but that's all.

→ええと, 私は日曜日にテニスをしました.

Well, I played tennis last Sunday.

→特に激しいことはなにもしていません.

I don't do anything particularly strenuous.

> strenuous：激しい, 非常に活発な

急性または亜急性のけが以外は保険が適用されません. それらは自己負担の診療（自由診療）で処置されます. よろしいですか.

Injuries other than acute and subacute injuries are not covered by insurance. They will be treated with treatments at your own expense. Is that OK?

> injuries other than 〜：〜以外のけが / insurance：保険 / at one's own expense：自己負担で

≡ けがに焦点を絞った患者の主訴表現

足を踏み外した拍子に足首を捻挫したようです.

When I slipped, I seem to have sprained my ankle.

> slip：足を踏み外す

バスケットボールをしていた時, 足首をねじってしまいました.

I twisted my ankle when I was playing basketball.

走った拍子に膝がガクンとなって，ものすごい痛みがありました．

I twisted my knee while running and it hurts terribly.

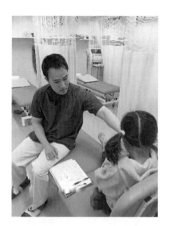

逆立ちをしていて，それから倒れました．

I was doing a handstand and then fell over.

`handstand：逆立ち / fall over：転ぶ`

テニスのラケットを振っていたら，突然背中がギクンとなりました．

When I was swinging my tennis racket, I suddenly felt my back pop.

`swing：振る / feel 〜 pop：〜がギクンとなるのを感じた`

棚の上の物を取ろうとしたら，突然背中にひどい痛みを感じました．

When I tried to get something off a high shelf, I suddenly felt a terrible pain shoot across my back.

`get 〜 off a shelf：棚から〜を取る / feel a pain shoot across 〜：〜に痛みが走るのを感じる`

One Point

けがの基本表現

ひねった：twisted / 〜に打ち身がある：have a bruise on 〜 / 突き指をした：jammed my finger, sprained my finger / 足首が腫れる：have a swollen ankle / 腫れた部分が熱をもっている：swollen area becomes warm / ぎっくり腰になった：strained my lower back / 腕を上げられません：can't lift my arm / 壁にぶつけた：run into a wall / ボールが当たった：I got hit with a ball / 〜と衝突した：be struck by 〜 / 自転車で転倒した：fell from one's bicycle / 手をついて転んだ：landed on one's hands / 頭（胸）を打った：hit one's head [chest] / しりもちをついた：fell on one's hip / 階段から落ちた：fell down the stairs /（段差などで）つまずいた：made a misstep / 横倒しに倒れた：fell sideways / 扉に挟んだ：got caught in the door

☰ 交通事故によるけが

ひょっとしたらそれは，先日の事故で，私たちの車が後ろからぶつけられた時のせいで起きたのかもしれません．

Perhaps it occurred because of the accident the other day when our car was hit from behind.

because of 〜：〜のせい / be hit from behind：後ろからぶつけられる

私が急ブレーキをかけた時に，首がガクンとなりました．／ 私が急ブレーキをかけた時に，むち打ち症になりました．

My neck snapped when I suddenly put on the brakes. / I had [got] whiplash when I suddenly put on the brakes.

put on the brakes：ブレーキを踏む / whiplash：むち打ち症

交通事故の場合は保険が異なります（違う保険が適用されます）．

Injuries caused by a traffic accident are covered by a different insurance program.

traffic accident：交通事故

☰ 痛みに焦点を絞った表現

（常に）痛みますか．

Does it hurt (all the time)?

→はい，時々とても鋭くなります．

Yes, it sometimes is very sharp.

→はい，でも少しは和らぎました．

Yes, but it seems to have lessened somewhat.

seem to 〜：〜するように思える / lessen：少なくなる / somewhat：ある程度，いくぶん

いつ頃から痛みが生じていますか．

When did the pain start?

その症状には最初にいつ気が付きましたか.

When did you first notice the symptoms? /
When was the first time you noticed the problem [symptom]?

first time you noticed ～：～に気づいた初めての時 / notice：気づく / symptom：症状

それは突然始まりましたか, それとも徐々に大きくなってきましたか.

Did it start suddenly or did it build up slowly?

build up：形成される

→痛みが始まったのは1～2週間前です.

The pain started a week or two ago.

→もうだいぶ前です.

It started long ago.

その痛みはどのくらいひどいのですか.

How severe is the pain?

かなり痛みますか.

Does it hurt much?

その痛みは激しいですか.

Is the pain severe?

→はい, とても我慢できません.

Yes, I can hardly bear the pain.

hardly：ほとんど～ない / bear：耐える

→最悪というわけではありません.

It's not too bad.

→我慢できないくらいとても激しいというものではありません.

It's not so severe that I can't put up with it.

so ～ that …：とても～なので…である

→とてもひどいというわけではありませんが, 時々不快感のせいで眠れません.

It's not too bad, but once in a while I can't sleep because of the discomfort.

once in a while：時々 / discomfort：不快感

→一時的に激痛がありましたが，今は少し和らぎました．

For a while it was very painful, but now it seems to have lessened somewhat.

for a while：しばらくの間

どこが痛むか，正確に教えてください．

Where exactly does it hurt?

exactly：正確に

痛むところを手で指し示してください．/
痛みを感じるところを指し示していただけますか．

**Show me where it hurts with your finger. /
Can you point to where you feel the pain?**

where it hurts：痛む場所 / where you feel pain：痛みを感じる場所

痛みを感じるのはどこですか．

Where do you feel the pain?

痛むところを見せてください．

Can you show me the painful area?

どのような痛みですか（どんな感じの痛みですか）．

**What is the pain like? / What does the pain feel like? /
What kind of pain is it?**

どんな痛みか説明してください．

Please describe the pain. / Can you describe the pain for me?

describe：説明する，描写する

One Point

痛みを表す表現

痛みを感じる：feel [have] (a) pain / ズキンズキンという痛み：throbbing pain /
焼けるような痛み：burning pain / 刺すような痛み：stabbing pain / 持続する痛み：continued pain

圧迫するような痛みですか.
Does it feel like pressure?

→痛いというより，こり固まった感じです.
It's not so much hurting, but more like a stiff feeling.
stiff：凝っている，固くなっている

触ると痛みますか.
Does it hurt when I touch it?

動かせますか.
Can you move it?

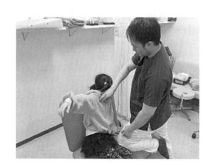

→少しなら動かせます.
I can move it just a little.

痛みはどこに広がりますか.
Where does the pain radiate?
radiate：広がる

どんな時に痛みますか（どうすれば痛みますか）.
What causes the pain?
cause：引き起こす

→この部分を動かすと痛いです.
When I move this part, it hurts.

→この部分を動かすと痛みが右足に走ります.
When I move this part, pain shoots to my right leg.
shoot：（痛みが）走る

→動かさなければ痛みません.
It doesn't hurt so long as I don't move.
so long as 〜：〜である限り

→膝を曲げると痛みます.
When I bend my knee, it hurts.

→首を動かそうとするとギクッとします.
When I try to turn my head, I feel a sharp pain.

sharp：激しい

→無理やり動かそうとするとすごく痛みます.
If I try to move it, it hurts terribly.

terribly：ひどく

→背中を伸ばそうとすると痛みます.
When I try to straighten my back, it hurts me.

straighten：まっすぐにする

One Point

〜すると痛い

動かすと痛い：It hurts when it moves / 押されると痛い：It hurts when pushed /
歩くと痛い：It hurts when walking / 座ると痛い：It hurts when sitting / 寝ると
痛い：It hurts when lying down / 荷重すると痛い：It hurts when weight is added

押すとどう感じますか.
When I press it, how does it feel?

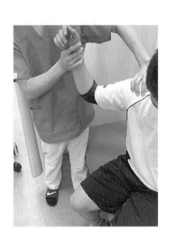

→ちょっと痛いです.
It hurts a little.

→押されると，飛び上がるほど痛いです.
When pushed or pressed, it hurts so much that I jump up [it makes me jerk].

なにをすると痛みますか.
What do you do when it hurts?

→歩くと左膝が痛みます.
When I walk, I feel pain in my left knee.

→いちばん痛むのは，朝起きる時です.
It hurts the most when I get up in the morning.

→朝と夕方が最悪です．

It's worst in the morning and the evening.

→昼間動いている時は，それほど気にならなくなります．

When I am moving about during the day, I often don't notice the pain.

> move about：動き回る

その痛みによる困難はなにかありますか．

Do you have any difficulties because of the pain?

> difficulty：困難

→右腕を伸ばすことができないので，家事をするのがたいへんです．

Because I can't stretch my right arm, I have trouble doing housework.

> stretch：伸ばす

→靴ひもを結ぶのに膝を曲げることができません．

I can't bend my knees to tie my shoelaces.

> bend：曲げる / shoelaces：靴ひも

→痛みのために自分の髪も自分でとかせません．

I can't comb my hair because of the pain.

> comb：（髪を）とかす

→仕事には特に影響しません．

It doesn't affect my ability to work in particular.

> affect：影響する / in particular：特に

≡ 痛みに焦点を絞った患者の主訴表現

右膝が痛いです．

I have a pain in my right knee.

肩と腕が痛みます．

My shoulders and arms hurt.

左肩が痛いです.
I feel a pain in my left shoulder.

左足首がすごく痛みます.
My left ankle hurts very much.

今朝起きたら, 首が痛くて. / 朝から首が痛くて.
**When I got up this morning, I had a crick in my neck. /
I have had a crick in my neck since this morning.**

crick：筋繊維を痛めてしまった状態

背中の下のほうがひどく痛みます. ここまで来るのがやっとでした.
**The lower part of my back hurts so terribly. I could hardly manage
to get here.**

can hardly manage to ～：なんとか～する

咳をすると, 背中のここが痛いです.
When I cough, my back hurts down here.

cough：咳をする

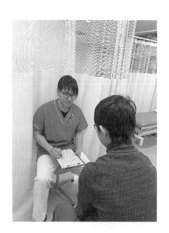

時々股関節が痛いのですが.
I sometimes have a pain in my thigh joints.

thigh joints：股関節

年齢の問題かもしれませんが, 左肩が凝って動かせません.
**It might be just a matter of age, but my left
shoulder is so stiff I can't move it.**

matter：問題

腕を上げたり, 曲げたりはできません.
I can't lift my arm or bend it.

lift：上げる

One
Point

患者に共感を示す表現

それはお気の毒に.　I'm sorry to hear that. / That's too bad.
よく分かります.　I understand.
それは困るでしょうね.　That sounds upsetting.

その他の症状

なにをすると楽になりますか.

What eases the pain?

どうすればひどくなったりよくなったりしますか.

Does anything make it worse or better?

make ～ worse (better)：～をより悪い（よい）状態にする

→マッサージすると, 少し楽に感じます.

If I massage it, it feels a little better.

→サポーターをすると, 少し楽に感じます.

If I wear a supporter, I feel a little more comfortable.

wear a supporter：サポーターを着ける / comfortable：快適な

→そこを湯に浸して温めると, 楽になります.

If I warm it by putting it in hot water, it feels better.

痛みの他に気になる症状はありますか.

Are there other symptoms that worry you besides the pain?

worry you：あなたを心配させる / besides ～：～の他に

→左足がしびれて, 歩くのに困難を感じます.

My left leg feels numb so it's hard to walk.

numb：しびれる

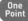

さまざまな症状の表現

腫れている：swollen / 熱感：burning sensation / 冷感：cool sensation / 動かない, 動けない：immovable / 力が入らない：ineffective / 曲がらない：does not bend

他にけがしたところや痛いところはありますか.
Do you have pain or an injury anywhere else?

> anywhere else：他のどこかに

→背中が少し痛いです.
My back hurts a little.

肩も痛みますか.
Do your shoulders hurt, too?

→肩も痛みます.
My shoulders hurt, too.

→それほどひどくありませんが，ちょっと痛みます.
It hurts, but not too much.

→打ち身のほうが痛くて，肩の痛みには気づきませんでした.
The bruise hurts more, so I didn't notice the shoulder.

腰や足はどうですか.
How about your hips or legs?

→それらはまったく大丈夫です.
They are quite all right.

→少し重たく感じますが，痛くありません.
They feel a little heavy, but they don't hurt.

≡ 職業

お仕事はどんなことをされていますか. / ご職業はなんですか.
What kind of work do you do? / What is your occupation?

ご職業をお聞きしてもよろしいですか.
May I ask what your occupation is?

→会社で経理をしています．
I am an accountant in a company.

accountant：経理担当者

→商社の営業部門にいます．
I'm in the sales department of a trading company.

sales department：営業部門 / trading company：商社

→技術者です．
I'm a technician.

→大学の講師です．
I'm a university teacher.

お勤め先はどちらですか．
Where do you work?

労災保険適用の場合

今回のけがは仕事中に起きたのですか．
Did the injury occur while you were working?

仕事中のけがであれば，施術に健康保険は適用されません．労災保険となります．
If the injury occurred while working, its treatment is not covered by health insurance. It will be covered by workers' compensation insurance.

workers' compensation insurance：労災保険

既往歴（past history / past medical history）

過去に大きな病気にかかったことはありますか．
Have you ever had any major illnesses before?

過去に大きなけがをしたことがありますか.

Have you ever been seriously injured in the past? / Have you ever had a serious injury in the past?

> seriously：ひどく / serious：ひどい

→いいえ，これまで大きなけがをしたことはありません.

No, I've never had any serious injuries.

過去に手術の経験はありますか.

Have you ever had an operation?

> operation：手術

体内に金属が埋め込まれていますか，たとえば，ペースメーカー，クリップ，髄内釘，人工関節などです.

Do you have any metal embedded in your body, such as a pacemaker, clip, intramedullary nail, artificial joint, and so on?

> metal：金属 / embed：埋め込む / intramedullary nail：髄内釘 / artificial joint：人工関節

患者が服用中の薬

普段飲まれている薬はありますか（なにか薬を飲んでいますか）.

Are you taking any medication?

> medication：薬剤，医薬

*Are you taking any drugs? は，「なにか麻薬をやっていますか」という意味にとられる可能性があるので避ける.

One Point

薬剤の英語

血栓阻害薬：thrombotic inhibitors / 鎮痛薬：analgesics / 抗うつ薬：antidepressants / 甲状腺関連薬：thyroid-related drugs / 糖尿病関連薬：diabetes-related drugs / 痛風関連薬：gout-related drugs / 抗リウマチ薬：anti-rheumatic drugs / 骨粗鬆症治療薬：osteoporosis drugs

他に私たちに話しておくような薬を飲んではいませんか.

Are you taking any other medication that we need to know about?

≡ その他

今回のけがに関して他の医療機関で治療中の場合，私たちから受ける施術に健康保険は適用されません．

If you are receiving treatment for the same injury at another medical institution, the treatment received from us is not covered by health insurance.

他に私が聞いておくべきことがありますか（なにか言い忘れたことがありますか）．

Is there anything else I should know?

他になにか質問はありますか．

Do you have any further questions?

further：さらなる

3 身体観察・評価のための表現

Expressions for the Physical Examination

Introduction

身体観察・評価も，適切な施術をするための判断材料を得るために必須です．本章では，実際に患部を観たり，触れたりするために必要な英語表現を学びます．身体に触れて調べること（palpation），患部（affected area），症状（symptom）などのキーワード，「うつ伏せになってください．」（Please lie on your stomach.），「ここを押すと痛みますか．」（Does it hurt when I press here?）のような重要表現がたくさんあります．

身体観察・評価の開始

身体観察をはじめます．

**Let's take a look (at you). / I'm going to examine you. /
I would like to examine you now. / May I take a look at you now? /
I will check your symptoms now.**

> examine：（患者の健康状態を）検査する（口語では look at で代替可能）

これから身体に触れて検査を始めます．

I will start the palpation now.

> palpation：身体に触れて調べること ＝ to examine 〜 by feeling with the hand

脱衣

服を脱いでください．/ 服を脱いでこのガウンに着替えてください．

Please take off your clothes. / Please disrobe and put on this gown.

> disrobe：服を脱ぐ（医師がよく使う動詞）

こちらの服に着替えてください．

Please change into these clothes.

上着（ズボン，スカート，靴下）を脱いでください．

Please take off your coat [trousers / skirts / socks].

スカートをまくり上げて，患部を見せてください．

Please lift up your skirt and show me the affected area.

lift up：（スカートを）まくり上げる

ズボンの裾をまくり上げてください．

Please roll up your trousers.

roll up：（裾を）まくり上げる

そでをまくってください．／そでをまくり上げて腕を見せてください．

Please pull up your sleeve. / Please roll up your sleeve so that I can see your arm.

pull up：（そでを）まくる / sleeve：そで（→本頁，One Point「服など身に着けるものに関する表現」） / so that ～ can …：～が…できるように

時計（眼鏡，アクセサリー）は外してください．

Please take off your watch [glasses / accessories].

ご用意ができましたらこちらの部屋にきてください．

Okay, once you get ready, please come to this room.

once ～：ひとたび～したら / ready：準備ができている

はい，準備ができました．

Yes, I'm ready.

One Point

服など身に着けるものに関する表現

服：clothes ／ シャツ：shirt ／ ズボン：pants, trousers ／ スカート：skirt ／ 上着：coat, jacket ／ 靴下：socks ／ そで：sleeve ／ 腕時計：watch ／ 眼鏡：glasses ／ アクセサリー：accessories ／ 指輪：ring

姿勢

立って（座って）ください．
Please stand up [sit down].

前（後ろ）を向いてください．
Please face the front [back].

face the front：前を向く / face the back：後ろを向く

右（左）を向いてください．
Please turn to your right [left] side.

turn to：〜のほうを向く（見る）

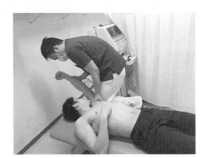

ベッドに上がって，仰向けに寝てください．
Hop onto the bed and lie on your back, please.

lie on one's back：仰向けになる / back：背中

うつ伏せになってください．
Please lie on your stomach.

lie on one's stomach：うつ伏せになる / stomach：腹部

右（左）を向いて寝てください．
Please lie down on your right [left] side.

lie down：寝ころぶ

こちらに座って，右腕（左足）をこのテーブル（フットレスト）に載せてください．
Please sit here and put your right arm [left leg] on this table [footrest].

私が「いいですよ」というまで動かないでください．
Please don't move until I say it's OK.

しばらく動かないでください．
Can you keep still for a while?

keep still：じっとしている

痛み

痛むところを見せてください.
Can you show me the painful area?

> painful area：痛む場所

じっとしていても痛みますか（安静時痛）.
Do you feel pain even if you remain still?

> pain：痛み / remain still：じっとしている

ここを触るとどう感じますか.
When I touch this point, how does it feel?

ここが固いですね.
This part [spot] is so stiff.

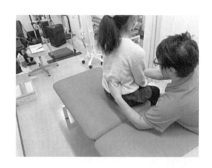

痛かったら教えてください.
If you feel pain, please let me know.

ここを押すと痛みますか.
Does it hurt when I press here?

→押されると痛いです.
It hurts when pushed.

> when pushed = when it is pushed

こちらに動かすと痛みますか.
Does it hurt when I move it this way?

→この部分を動かすと痛いです.
When I move this part, it hurts.

→動かさなければ痛みません.
It doesn't hurt so long as I don't move.

> so long as 〜：〜である限り

この部分を曲げると痛みますか.
Does it hurt if you bend here?

この部分を伸ばすと痛みますか.

Does it hurt when you stretch this part?

運動

私と同じ動きをしてみてください.

Can you do the same movement as I do? /

（動作を示しながら）**Please do this.**

> the same movement as 〜：〜するのと同じ動き

私の動かす方向と反対方向に，右腕に力をいれてください.

Use the strength in your right arm to push in the direction opposite to mine.

> in the direction opposite to 〜：〜とは反対方向に

押し返してください.

Please push back.

右腕（肘，腰，足，膝，足首）を伸ばして（曲げて）ください.

Can you stretch out [bend] your right arm [elbow / waist / leg / knee / ankle]?

右腕（肩，肘，腰，足，膝，足首）がどのくらい動くか見せてください.

Can you show me how well you can move your right arm [shoulder / elbow / waist / leg / knee / ankle]?

右腕（肩，ひじ，腰，足，膝，足首）に関して何が問題ですか.

What problems do you have with your right arm [shoulder / elbow / waist / leg / knee / ankle]?

→無理やり動かそうとすると，すごく痛みます.

If I try to make it move, it hurts terribly.

≡ 呼吸

息を吸って（吐いて）ください．/ 息を止めてください．
Please breathe in [breathe out]. / Please hold your breath.

> breathe in：息を吸う / breathe out：息を吐く / breath：息，呼吸

深呼吸してください．
Please take a deep breath.

≡ 身体観察の終了

はい，終了しました．
Okay, it's done.

楽にしてください．
Please relax.

気分は悪くないですか．
Are you OK? / Do you feel sick?

服を着てください．/ 服を着ていただいて結構です．
Please put your clothes back on. / You can get dressed now.

> put ～ back on：脱いだものを再び着る / get dressed：服を着た状態になる

そのまま少しお待ちください．
Please wait just for a moment.

4 評価の告知のための表現
Expressions for the Examination Results

Introduction

本章では，医療面接，身体観察に基づいた判断を患者に伝えるための表現を学びます．打撲（contusion），損傷（injury），骨折（fracture）などの傷病名，「太ももの肉離れです．」（You have a thigh muscle strain.）のような必須表現を確認しましょう．さらに，他の医療機関への紹介の必要がある場合の「医院あるいは病院への紹介状を書きます．」（I will write a referral letter to a clinic or hospital.）のような表現も重要な学習事項です．

捻挫

これは捻挫です．/ 足首を捻挫しています．
This is a sprain. / You have a sprained ankle.

> **sprained ankle：捻挫した足首**

打撲・筋挫傷

これは打撲です．
This is a bruise.

靭帯の損傷です．/ 膝の靭帯の損傷です．
You have a ligament injury. / You have a damaged ligament of the knee.

> **ligament：靭帯（→ p35, One Point「主な組織名」）**

筋挫傷の可能性が強いですが，断裂しているかもしれません．
The possibility of a muscle contusion is strong, but it may be ruptured.

> **be ruptured：断裂している**

肉離れです. / 太ももの肉離れです.

You have a pulled muscle. / You have a thigh muscle strain.

pulled muscle, muscle strain：肉離れ（→ p35，One Point「主な傷病・症状」）

脱臼

肩が脱臼しています. / 脱臼しています.

Your shoulder is dislocated. / You have a dislocation.

be dislocated：脱臼している / dislocation：脱臼（→ p35，One Point「主な傷病・症状」）

関節の状態からみて, 脱臼しています.

Judging from its state, you have a dislocated joint.

judging from 〜：〜から判断して

骨折

たぶん骨折しています.

The bone is probably fractured.

be fractured：骨折している

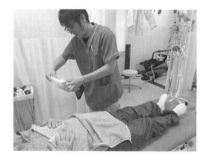

骨折しているかもしれません.

**The bone may be fractured. /
Maybe the bone is fractured. /
Perhaps, the bone is fractured.**

ひょっとすると骨折しているかもしれません.

The bone is possibly fractured.

 One Point

「たぶん」「かもしれない」可能性, 確信を表す副詞

病院での診療を強く勧めるくらい可能性が高いなら **probably**
本当に五分五分で念のため病院での受診を勧めるなら **maybe** か **perhaps**
確信はないが可能性として考えておかなければならない程度なら **possibly**

不全骨折の可能性があります.

**It may be an insufficiency fracture. /
There may be an insufficiency fracture (in the bone / here).**

`insufficiency fracture：不全骨折`

ここは, 疲労骨折を起こしているかもしれません.

It may be a stress fracture. / There may be stress fractures here.

`stress fracture：疲労骨折 / be stress fractured：疲労骨折になっている`

捻挫しているようにみえますが, 裂離骨折の可能性が否定できません.

**It seems to be a sprain, but the possibility of an avulsion fracture
cannot be denied.**

`possibility：可能性 / avulsion fracture：裂離骨折 / deny：否定する`

One Point

主な組織名

骨：bone / 関節：joint / 筋 (肉)：muscle / 腱：tendon / 靱帯：ligament / 神経：
nerve / 血管：blood vessel / 皮下組織：subcutaneous tissue

One Point

主な傷病・症状

骨折：fracture / ひび割れ：crack / 脱臼：dislocation / 打撲, 挫傷：contusion,
bruise / 捻挫：sprain / 損傷：injury / 肉離れ：pulled muscle, muscle strain / 断
裂：rupture / 炎症：inflammation / ヘルニア：hernia / 首のこり：stiff neck / 肩
こり：stiff shoulder / 腰痛・ぎっくり腰：lower back strain / 突き指：sprained
finger / むち打ち：neck strain, whiplash

他の医療機関への紹介

レントゲン写真で骨の状態を確認する必要があります．診療所あるいは病院への紹介状を書きます．

You need an X-ray of your bone. So, I will write a referral letter to a clinic or hospital.

かかりつけの病院はありますか（医師はいますか）．

Do you have a family hospital [local GP / primary care doctor]?

> family hospital：かかりつけの病院 / local GP：地域の総合診療医（GP = general physician）／
> primary care doctor：かかりつけの医師

痛みや症状が内臓疾患由来，あるいは精神疾患由来の可能性がある場合

この痛みは，けが以外の原因からもたらされている可能性があります．

This pain may be caused by a factor other than injury.

> be caused by ～：～によって引き起こされる / factor other than injury：けが以外の要因

けがの痛みではないので，私たちは治療できません．

It is not a pain caused by injury, so we cannot treat it.

内科の受診をお勧めします．

I recommend that you see an internal medicine doctor.

> recommend that someone ～：（人が）～することを勧める / internal medicine：内科

精神科の受診をお勧めします．

I recommend that you see a psychiatrist. /
I recommend that you visit a psychiatric hospital.

> psychiatrist：精神科医 / psychiatric hospital：精神科医院

5 施術開始時，施術中の汎用的表現
Common Expressions for Treatment Procedures

Introduction

本章では，さまざまな施術において共通に使われる汎用的表現を提示します．施術は treatment あるいは therapy といいます．「今日の体の調子はいかがですか．」(How are you feeling today?) のような定型表現，「患部の動きを確認しましょう．」(Let me check the movement of the affected area.)，「痛いところを触りますよ．」(I will touch the painful area.) などのような必須表現を覚えましょう．

施術開始時

これから施術をしていきます．
I will start the treatment now. / I will begin the therapy now.

今日の体の調子はいかがですか．/ ご様子はいかがですか．
How are you feeling today?

前回の状態と比べてどうですか．
How are you feeling today compared to the last time we met?

the last time we met：前回私たちが会った時

けがの具合はいかがですか．
How is your injury (coming along)?

coming along：よくなる，うまくいく

腕（首，膝，足首）の具合はいかがですか．
How is your arm [neck / knee / ankle] (coming along) ?

施術を始める前に，患部の動きを確認しましょう．

Before starting the treatment, let me check the movement of the affected area. /
Before starting the therapy, can you show me how well you can move the affected area?

how well you can 〜：どのくらいよく〜できるか

痛いところを触りますよ．

I will touch the painful area.

施術中

この体勢はつらくないですか．

Is it hard to keep this posture [position]?

keep this posture：この姿勢を保つ

ここが固いですね．

This part [spot] is so stiff.

大丈夫ですか．痛くないですか．

Are you OK? Do you feel pain [Is it painful]?

もし痛いようでしたら言ってください．

If you feel pain, please let me know.

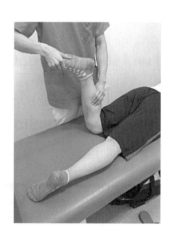

整復の施術のための表現
Expressions for Reduction Treatment

Introduction

「(けがをした部位を) 整復する」を表す医学英語は, reposition, reduce の 2 つが使われていますが, 整形外科学の学術文献では通例, reduce が使用されています. reduce は, 日常語では「減らす」を意味しますが, ラテン語の reduco (re=後ろへ, duco=戻す) が語源であることを知れば, 不思議はないですね. 患肢 (affected limb) のようなキーワード,「痛みを伴うこがありますが, 処置後は楽になります.」(It may be painful, but you will feel better after the procedure.) のような重要表現を確認してください.

整復で共通にかける言葉

これから整復を始めます.

I will start the reduction now.

reduction：整復

整復とは, 骨折や脱臼した骨を元の位置に戻すことです.

Reduction is to reposition bones to their normal position after a fracture or dislocation.

reposition：元の場所に戻す

これまでに整復を受けたことはありますか.

Have you ever received reduction treatment?

→ありません. 初めてです. / はい, あります. 2回目です.

No, I haven't. This is my first time. / Yes, I have. This is my second time.

整復は痛みを伴うことがありますが, 処置後は楽になります.

Reduction treatment may cause pain [It may be painful], but you will feel better after the procedure.

procedure：処置

数回の整復操作が必要となる場合があります.

Several operations may be performed. / You may undergo multiple operations.

undergo：経験する

痛みを我慢できない時は，教えてください.

If it is too painful [If you cannot stand the pain, If you cannot endure the pain], please let me know.

stand, endure：耐える，我慢する

手をあげて知らせてください.

Please let me know by raising your hand. / Please raise your hand to let me know.

raise：あげる

どこかを軽く叩いて知らせてください.

Please let me know by tapping anywhere.

tap：軽く叩く

整復中，気分が悪くなったりした場合は，言ってください.

If you get sick during the reduction [reduction treatment, treatment, procedure], please let me know.

get sick：気分が悪くなる

気分が悪くなったら，中止します.

If you get sick, I will stop the operation [treatment].

整復するため，患部に触ります.

I will touch the affected area in order to reduce it.

すみませんが，少し痛みます.

I'm sorry, but it will be slightly painful.

slightly：わずかに

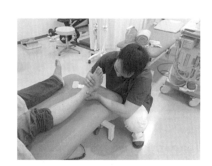

痛いですが，我慢してください.

It will be painful, but please be patient.

patient：（形容詞）忍耐強い

少しの間我慢してください.

Please be patient for a moment [while].

for a moment：少しの間

（なるべく）力を抜いてください．

Please relax (as much as possible).

as much as possible：できるだけ

呼吸を止めないでください．/ なるべく息を止めないでください．

Remember to keep breathing.

breathing：呼吸

ゆっくりと呼吸し続けてください．/ ゆっくりと息を吸って，吐いてください．

Please keep breathing slowly. / Please breathe in and out slowly.

breath out：息を吐く

ゆっくりと患肢を牽引します．/ ゆっくりと患肢を引っ張ります．

OK. I will now slowly apply a traction force to the affected limb. / OK. I will now pull the affected bone slowly.

apply：適用する / traction force：牽引力 / affected limb：患肢

痛いですか．

Does it hurt?

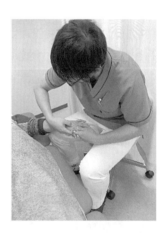

骨がよい位置まで戻ってきています．

It is now in a good position. / It is close to the normal position.

normal position：正常な位置

もう少し我慢できますか．/ 頑張ってください．

Please be patient for a little while longer.

a little while longer：あともう少しの間

もう終わります．

It is almost done.

整復後は指示するまで動かないでください．/ 私が「いいですよ」というまで動かないでください．

After the reduction, please don't move until I say it's OK.

until 〜：〜するまで

はい，できました．

Okay, it's done.

これで整復が終わりました.
The reduction is done. / The reduction treatment is finished.

よく頑張りました.
Thank you for your patience [cooperation].

> patience：忍耐 / cooperation：協力

左右同じになりました（元の位置に戻りました）.
Now, it is in the normal position.

患部が炎症を起こしていますので, 冷却します.
Since the affected area is inflamed, I will cool it down.

> be inflamed：炎症を起こしている / cool 〜 down：〜を冷やす

冷たすぎませんか.
Is it too cold?

（整復の）後は患部を固定していきます.
Next, I will immobilize the affected area.

> immobilize：固定する

骨折の整復

骨折していますので, 整復をします.
The bone is fractured [The bone is broken / You have a fracture], so I will reduce it.

> bone is fractured, bone is broken：骨折している /（人，動物）have a fracture：骨折している / reduce：整復する

〈完全骨折〉
今から, 折れてずれた骨を元の位置に戻します. / ずれている骨の位置を合わせます.
I will reposition the displaced bone to its normal position.

> displaced bone：ずれた骨

〈剥離骨折, 裂離骨折（avulsion fracture）〉
はがれた骨片を元の位置に戻します.

I will reposition the fragment to its normal position.

> fragment：一片, 断片

〈若木骨折（greenstick fracture）〉
曲がった骨を元の状態に戻します.

I will return the bent bone to its normal shape.

> bent：曲げられた（←bend：曲げる）

〈転位のない骨折（non-displaced fracture）〉
骨は折れていますが整復の必要はありません.

The bone is fractured, but reduction is not necessary.

骨片の転位がないので, 整復の必要はありません.

Since the bone fragments are not displaced, reduction is not necessary.

脱臼

脱臼しているので, 整復をします.

You have a dislocation, so I will reduce [fix] it. / The joint is dislocated, so I will reduce [reposition] it.

> have a dislocation：（人, 動物が）脱臼している / fix：元に戻す, 整復する / joint is dislocated：関節が脱臼している

初めて肩（腕）を脱臼したのはいつ頃ですか.

When did you first dislocate your shoulder [arm]?

自分で肩を脱臼させることはできますか.

Can you dislocate your shoulder by yourself?

これから腕（足, 指）を動かして（引っ張って）, 骨を関節の正しい位置に戻します.

I will move [pull] the dislocated arm [leg / finger] and reduce it into its normal position. / I will move [pull] the dislocated arm [leg / finger] and return it into its normal position.

> pull：引っ張る, 引く

≡ その他

このような関節の状態の場合，あなたは患部を牽引してはいけません．

When the joint is in this state, you must not pull the affected part.

state：状態

錘と重力を使って整復します．

I will reduce it by using weight and gravity.

weight：錘 / gravity：重力

固定の施術のための表現
Expressions for Immobilization Treatment

Introduction

固定では，患者とコミュニケーションをとりながら施術をしていきます．「力を抜いてください．」(Please relax.)，「この範囲を固定していきます．」(I will immobilize this area.)，「きつくないですか．」(Is it too tight?)，「痛い時は，おっしゃってください．」(If it hurts, please let me know.) などの表現は基本です．また，「痛いところが出たらすぐに電話で連絡してください．」(If pain occurs, please call me.) のようなフォローアップのための表現も覚えましょう．

固定で共通にかける言葉

無事整復できましたので，患部を固定します．

The reduction is done. Now, I will immobilize the affected area. / The reduction treatment is over. Now, I will secure the affected area.

secure：固定する

固定は，損傷部位の整復された位置を維持します．

Immobilization maintains the reduced position of the injured area.

immobilization：固定 / reduced position：整復された位置

温めると軟らかくなり，冷めると硬くなる材料を使います．

I will use a material which becomes soft when heated and hard when cooled.

material which becomes soft：軟らかくなる材料 / when heated = when it is heated：温められた時 / and hard when cooled = becomes hard when it is cooled：冷まされた時に硬くなる

固定をしていきます．

I will start the immobilization process. / I will secure the affected area.

process：処置

この固定材料は，保険の適用外となります．

This immobilization material is not covered by health insurance.

力を抜いてください．

Please relax.

この範囲を固定していきます．

I will immobilize this area.

固定中は患肢を動かさないでください．

Please don't move the injured limb during the immobilization procedure.

limb：手足

気分が悪くなったら，中止します．

If you feel sick, I will stop the procedure.

sick：具合が悪い

痛い時（熱い時）は言ってください．

If it hurts [If it's too hot], please let me know.

また，固定がきついと感じるようでしたら言ってください．

Also, if it's too tight, please let me know.

tight：きつい

きつく（緩く）ないですか（窮屈過ぎないですか，苦しくないですか）．/ 緩くないですか．

Is it too tight [loose]?

loose：緩い

固定がしびれや麻痺を生じさせることがあります．

The mobilization may cause numbness or paralysis in your injured limb.

numbness：しびれ / paralysis：麻痺

関節が固まらないように動かせる部分から動かしていきます．

In order to prevent the joint from stiffening, I will move the other movable parts.

prevent 〜 from …ing：〜が…することを防ぐ / joint：関節（→ p35, One Point「主な組織名」）/ stiffening：固くなること / movable：動かすことが可能な

固定中は患肢を動かさないでください.

Please don't move the injured limb during the immobilization procedure.

固定している範囲以外の関節は動かすようにしてください.

Please move the joints that are not immobilized.

固定している関節は動かせませんが, 指は動かすようにしてください.

You cannot move the immobilized joint, but please move your fingers.

固定してないところは動かすようにしてください. 拘縮の予防となります.

Please try to move your body parts that are not immobilized. It will prevent contracture.

> contracture：拘縮

ギプス（cast）

ギプスで患部を固定します.

**I will immobilize the injured area with a cast. / I will put the injured area in a cast. /
I will set the injured area in a cast.**

> cast：ギプス（gips,「石膏」を意味するドイツ語）

ギプスは少し重たいと感じますが, 皮膚を傷つけることは少ないです.

You might feel that the cast is a bit heavy, but it rarely hurts the skin.

> a bit：少し / rarely：ほとんど～ない

患部をギプスで押さえる時に（固定する時に）, 少し痛いかもしれません.

It may slightly hurt when the injured area is immobilized with a cast.

ギプスが固まるまで少し時間がかかります.

It takes some time for the material to harden [set].

> it takes … for ～ to ―：～が―するのに（時間が）…くらいかかる / harden = set：固くなる

固定材（ギプス）が固まるまで動かないでください.

Please don't move the injured limb until the material hardens [sets].

大丈夫ですか.

Are you OK?

これで固定ができました.

OK, the immobilization is done.

固定によって，痛みを感じるところはありますか.

Are there any painful spots due to the immobilization?

due to 〜：〜のせいで

→今は大丈夫です.

I'm OK now.

最後に血液循環の確認をします.

Finally, I will check your blood circulation.

blood circulation：血液循環

≡ ギプス固定後

固定がきつくて，当たって痛いところはないですか.

Do you feel (a) pain due to the tightness?

tightness：きついこと

しびれはありませんか.

Do you have any numbness in the injured limb?

固定がしびれや麻痺を生じさせることがあります.

The mobilization may cause numbness or paralysis in your injured limb.

腫れが増す時，固定がきつくなり過ぎる場合があります.

If the swelling increases, it may get too tight.

swelling：腫れ

血流が止まる感じや，しびれ，痛み，感覚異常がでるようであれば，その時は外せるなら外してよいです（すぐに連絡をしてください）．

If you feel that you have poor blood flow, numbness, pain, or abnormalities in sensation, you can take it off [please let me know].

poor blood flow：血行が悪い / abnormalities in sensation：感覚異常 / take 〜 off：外す

締め付けが強すぎる時はすぐに固定を外してください．

If it is too tight, please take it off.

経過がよければ，2週間くらいでギプスを外すことができます．

If you improve, we can take the cast off in about two weeks.

if you improve：経過がよければ

→それまでギブスをはめたままなのですね．

Until then do I have to wear this cast?

→一日中していなければいけないのですか．

Do I have to wear the support all day long?

不自由でしょうが，1〜2週間我慢してください．

It won't be convenient, but you will have to put up with it for a week or two.

put up with：我慢する

帰宅して違和感が生じたらすぐに連絡をください．

If you feel something is wrong after getting home, please let me know.

feel something is wrong：違和感が生じる

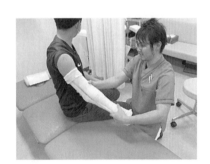

痛いところが出たらすぐに電話で連絡してください．

If pain occurs, please call me.

これが携帯電話の番号です．

This is my cell phone number.

≡ シーネ (splint)

シーネ*で患部を固定します.
I will immobilize the injured area with a splint.

*シーネは副木を意味するドイツ語 (schiene).

シーネは,患部を固定するために使われる固定材です.
A splint is a device used to immobilize an injured area.

`device：材料, 装置`

ギプス固定と比べてシーネ固定のほうが圧倒的に軽いです.
Compared to casts, splints are much lighter.

`compared to 〜：〜と比べて / much lighter：ずっと軽い (much + 比較級)`

巻いている最中に,少し温かさを感じると思います.
While the splint is being applied, you will feel a slight sense of warmth.

`warmth：暖かさ`

熱かったり,怖い感じがあったら教えてください (キャストカット時).
If it is too hot, or if you are afraid, please let me know.

熱く感じることがありますが,すぐに収まります.
It might feel hot, but it will subside soon.

`subside：なくなる, 治る`

すぐに固まります.
It will soon harden [set].

腫れて痛くなったり,きつくなったりしたら,すぐに連絡をください.
If the swelling increases, causing pain or tightness, please let me know.

包帯

包帯で患部を固定します.

I will immobilize the injured area using bandages.

bandage：包帯

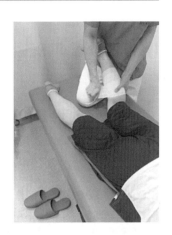

テーピングと違って, 包帯は肌にやさしいです.

Unlike taping, bandages are gentle to your skin.

unlike〜：〜と違って

血の流れが悪いと感じる時は, ためらわず（すぐに）外してください.

If you feel that you have poor blood flow, please don't hesitate to take it off.

hesitate to〜：〜することをためらう

（患部が足首の場合）立った時に違和感はありませんか.

Does something feel wrong when you stand up?

今日は包帯を外さないでください.

Please do not take off the bandages today.

包帯を外したら, 次回この包帯を持ってきてください.

If you take off the bandages, please bring them next time.

→この包帯はいつになったら取れるのですか.

When can I take off this bandage?

少しよくなったらサポーターに変えますから, それまで我慢してください.

When it's a little better, we will change to a support, so just be a little patient.

テーピング

テープを使って患部を固定します.
I will immobilize the injured area by using tape.

テーピングは,負傷した身体部分を固定または安定させるのに役立ちます.
Taping can help immobilize or stabilize an injured body part.

> stabilize：安定させる

皮膚がつっぱって痛くないですか（つっぱる感じで痛みはありませんか）.
Do you feel pain in your skin due to the tape's pulling sensation or stickiness?

> pulling sensation：つっぱる感じ,引っ張られる感じ

固定したうえ（状態）でお風呂に入るのは大丈夫です.
You can take a bath after securing the injured part.

テープは皮膚に直接巻きますか.
Would you like to place the tape directly on your skin?

皮膚に直接巻く際に,粘着剤等で皮膚がかぶれることがあります.
If tape is applied [If you wear tape] directly on your skin, skin irritation may occur due to the adhesive.

> wear tape：テープを巻く,テープを貼る / irritation：かぶれ / adhesive：粘着剤

皮膚はかぶれやすいですか.
Is your skin easily irritated? / Do you have sensitive skin that tends to get irritated?

> get irritated：かぶれる

テープを（貼るテンションを）強めに巻きますか.
Would you like me to wrap tape tightly? / Would you like the taping applied tightly?

> would like 〜 to …：〜（人）に…してほしい / wrap：（他者の身体に）テープを巻く（貼る）/ tightly：きつく / would like 〜 applied：適用された〜を望む（would like 〜 過去分詞）

かゆみは（かゆく）ありませんか.
Do you feel an itching sensation? / Do you have an itch?

> itching (sensation)：かゆみ

この部位は毛を剃る必要があります.

This body part needs to be shaved.

shave：（毛を）剃る

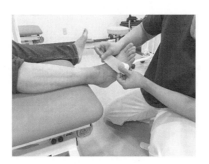

≡ サポーター類

医療用サポーター類は患部を守ることができます.

Medical supporters can protect an injured area.

まず私がつけ方をお見せしますので，その後にご自身でつけてみましょう.

I will show you how to put the supporter on. Then please try to put the supporter on by yourself.

正しいつけ方でつけてください.

Please put on and wear the supporter properly.

properly：適切に

お風呂などで外したらまた着けていてください.

Don't forget to put it on again after taking a bath.

強く締め付けすぎないように気をつけてください.

Please be careful not to fasten the supporter too tightly.

be careful not to 〜：〜しないように気をつける

≡ その他

固定材を止めるために，ご自身で巻ける伸びる包帯を持ち帰ってください（お渡しておきます）．

Please take elastic bandages back home with you so that you can secure the immobilization material by yourself. /
Please take elastic bandages back home with you. With these bandages, you can secure the immobilization material by yourself.

elastic bandage：伸縮包帯 / immobilization material：固定材

健側で副子を成形します（健側をモデルにして副子を成形します）．

I will make a splint using the unaffected limb as a model.

splint：副子 / unaffected limb：けがをしていない手足

保険の範囲（適用）内での固定を希望されますか．

Would you like an immobilization method that is covered by health insurance?

immobilization method：固定方法

この厚紙は医療用の固定材料です．

This cardboard is fixation material for medical use.

cardboard：厚紙 / fixation：固定

この金属副子は保険の対象です．

This metal splint is covered by health insurance.

metal splint：金属副子（金網副子は ladder splint）

この三角巾はなるべく外さないでください（どうしても外す必要がある場合を除いて，外さないでください）．

Please do not take off this sling unless it's really necessary.

sling：三角巾 / unless 〜：〜である場合以外

8 物理療法の施術のための表現

Expressions for Physical Therapy

物理療法の施術では，「～療法は，痛みを緩和する効果が望めます.」（～ therapy has pain-relieving effects.）のように，施術の効果を説明することは必須ですが，施術によって起こる可能性のあるリスクを回避するための配慮がさらに重要です.「体内に金属性のものはありませんか.」（Do you have anything metallic in your body?）のような，重要表現がいくつもあります. また,「ピリピリ感じるでしょう」（You will feel a tingling sensation.）のように刺激の感じ方を表す英語表現も確認してください.

物理療法で共通にかける言葉

体内にペースメーカーが（は）入っていませんか.
Do you have a pacemaker in your body?

妊娠の可能性はありませんか.
Is there any chance that you may be pregnant? / Are you currently pregnant?

pregnant：妊娠している

今までにステントを入れる手術を受けていませんか. /
体内にステントが入っていませんか.
Have you ever had an operation to place a stent in your body? / Do you have a stent in your body?

place：置く，入れる / stent：ステント

※ステント：人体の管状の部分（血管，気管，尿道など）を管腔内部から広げる医療機器で，多くの場合，金属でできた筒状のもの.

人工関節やプレート，ワイヤーなど体内に金属性のものはありませんか.
Do you have anything metallic in your body, such as an artificial joint, plate, or wire?

metallic：金属性の

過去に電気療法で気分が悪くなったことがありませんか.

Have you ever gotten sick due to electric therapy before?

electric therapy：電気療法

この療法の所要時間は15〜20分です.

It takes 15-20 minutes. / This therapy procedure takes 15-20 minutes.

この物理療法は健康保険の対象外となります

This physical therapy is not covered by health insurance.

physical therapy：物理療法

刺激が強すぎたり熱すぎたりしたら教えてください.

If the stimulation is too strong or too hot, please let me know.

stimulation：刺激

刺激がちょうどいいところで教えてください.

When the stimulation feels strong but comfortable, please let me know.

刺激を感じたら教えてください.

When you start to feel the stimulation, please let me know.

痛みはないですか.

Do you feel pain?

異常を感じたらすぐに教えてください.

If something feels wrong, please let me know immediately.

immediately：すぐに

施術中に気分が悪くなった場合は，言ってください.

If you feel sick during the treatment [therapy procedure], please let me know.

緊急の場合はここを押すと停止します.

In case of an emergency, press this button. It will stop the procedure.

痛みや温度変化に対して感覚が鈍くなる病気*はありませんか.

Do you have a disease that reduces your ability to feel pain or temperature changes?

> disease：病気, 疾患 / reduce：減らす / ability to ～：～する能力 / temperature：温度

*痛みや温度変化に対して感覚が鈍くなる病気としては, 糖尿病性ニューロパチー (diabetic peripheral neuropathy) などがある.

この療法は, 感覚のないところには使用することができません（痛みや熱を感じない部位には使用できません）.

This therapy cannot be applied to body parts that don't feel pain or heat.

> be applied：適用される / body parts that don't ～：～しない部位

低周波療法

（これから）低周波療法を行います.

Let's begin the low-frequency current therapy now.

> low-frequency current therapy：低周波療法

低周波療法は, 微弱な電気を人体に加えることによって, 痛みを和らげる物理療法です.

Low-frequency current therapy is a method of physical therapy which relieves pain by applying a weak electric current to the human body.

> relieve pain：痛みを和らげる / weak electric current：弱い電流

低周波療法は, 慢性的な痛みやしびれの症状に効果があります.

Low-frequency therapy is effective for chronic pain and numbness.

周波数や極性により感じ方が変わります.

You will feel differently depending on the frequency and polarity.

> depending on ～：～しだいで / frequency：周波数 / polarity：極性

ピリピリと感じます（ピリピリと感じるでしょう）.

You will feel a tingling sensation.

> tingling sensation：ピリピリとした感じ

ピリピリと感じてきたら教えてください.

When you feel a tingling sensation, please let me know.

刺激の強さはこれくらいで大丈夫でしょうか. 強すぎますか. 弱すぎますか.

How do you feel about the stimulation intensity at the moment? Is it too strong, or too low?

intensity：強さ

最初は少し弱いと感じるくらいで大丈夫です.

When it starts, it is normal to feel low stimulation intensity.

痛みを感じる前に刺激量を増やすのを止めます　痛みを感じたら言ってください

I will stop increasing [I will control] the intensity of stimulation before you feel pain. So, if you feel pain, please let me know.

痛くない範囲で, 刺激をしっかり感じたら教えてください.

Once you start to feel intense stimulation in a strong but comfortable range, please let me know.

干渉波，中周波

干渉波療法を行います.

Let's start the interferential current therapy now.

interferential current therapy：干渉波療法

これは電気治療の一種です. 干渉波を用いて身体を刺激します.

This is a type of electric therapy. It stimulates an area of your body using stimulation called interferential currents.

a type of ～：一種の～

干渉波療法は, 深部の筋肉組織に作用し, 疼痛を緩解します.

Interferential current therapy acts on deeper muscle tissues and relieves pain.

act on ～：～に作用する / deeper muscle tissues：深部の筋肉組織

少しの間この吸引導子の跡が肌につきますが, 気になりませんか.

You will have some vacuum electrode marks on your skin for a while. Are you OK with that [Does that bother you]?

vacuum electrode mark：吸引導子の跡

自動で周波数が切り換ります．
The frequency will change automatically.

automatically：自動的に

≡ 超音波

超音波療法を行います．
Let's start the ultrasound therapy now.

ultrasound therapy：超音波療法

超音波の振動刺激が患部の深部を温めます．
Ultrasonic vibration stimulus warms the deeper part of the affected area.

ultrasonic vibration stimulus：超音波の振動刺激 / warm：温める

この刺激は，血流を増加させます．
It increases the blood flow.

blood flow：血流

超音波の振動刺激は，腫れ，炎症および痛みを軽減します．
Ultrasonic vibration stimuli reduce swelling, inflammation, and pain.

stimuli：刺激（stimulus）の複数形

超音波の振動刺激は，治癒を促進します（超音波の振動刺激で患部が早くよくなります）．
Ultrasonic vibration stimulus promotes healing.

promote：促進する / healing：治癒

患部が温められます．
The injured area will be warmed up.

熱いと感じたら教えてください．/ 熱すぎませんか．
If it is too hot, please let me know. / Is it too hot?

患部に低音が響くような感覚を受けることがあります．
You may feel as if a low pitch sound is echoing in the affected area.

as if ～：まるで～であるように / low pitch sound：低音 / echo：響く

ジェルが塗ってありますので，少しぬるっと（ぬるぬる）します．

Since gel is used, it will feel a little greasy.

gel：ジェル / greasy：ぬるぬるした

ゆっくりと円を描くように，プローブを動かし続けてください．

Please keep moving the probe in slow and circular movements.

probe：プローブ / circular movement：円を描くような動き

皮膚の同じ場所にプローブを置き続けないでください．

Please do not keep placing the probe on the same place on your skin.

keep placing 〜：〜を置き続ける

プローブはゆっくりでよいので常に動かし続けてください（絶えず移動させてください）．

You don't have to move the probe fast, but please keep moving it.

プローブの移動を止めると危険です．

If you stop the movement, it is dangerous.

止めてしまうと音波痛が生じることがあります．

If you stop the movement, the ultrasound may cause pain.

患部に痛みを感じたら教えてください．

If you feel pain in the affected area, please let me know.

水分（ジェル）が不足すると効果が伝わりません．

If the gel dries up, the waves are not transmitted and there is no effect.

dry up：乾く / transmit：伝える

中周波療法，高周波療法

高周波療法を行います．

Let's start the high-frequency current therapy now.

high-frequency current therapy：高周波療法

高周波療法は，微弱な電気を人体に加えることによって，痛みを和らげる物理療法です．

High-frequency current therapy is a method of physical therapy which relieves pain by applying a weak electric current to the human body.

高周波療法は，筋肉の奥深い部分まで作用して，急性の痛みやこりを緩和します．

High-frequency current therapy works deep into the muscles and relieves acute pain and stiffness.

急速に熱くなることがあります．すぐに教えてください．

Sometimes it gets too hot quite rapidly. In such a case, please let me know immediately.

> rapidly：急速に

通電部にクリームを塗る必要があります．

It is necessary to apply cream to the current-carrying part.

> current-carrying part：通電部

温浴

温浴療法を行います．

Let's start the warm bath therapy now.

> warm bath therapy：温浴療法

温浴療法では，患部を温水に浸してもらいます．

In warm bath therapy, you are required to soak the injured area in hot water.

> be required to ～：～することを求められる / soak：浸す

温浴療法は血流を改善し，治癒を促進します．

Warm bath therapy increases the blood flow and promotes healing.

患部が温水で温められ，気泡が軽いマッサージ効果をもたらしてくれます．

The hot water warms the affected area and the bubbles produce a light massage effect.

> bubble：気泡，泡 / massage effect：マッサージ効果

腕（足）を温水に入れてください．
Please soak your arm [foot] in the hot water.

お湯のなかに患部を入れていきます．
I will place the injured area in the hot water.

患側をお湯のなかに入れてください．
Please soak the affected side in the hot water.

患部を温めてから運動療法を行います．
After warming the affected area, we will start the exercise therapy.

`exercise therapy：運動療法`

牽引

牽引療法を行います．
Let's start traction therapy now.

`traction therapy：牽引療法`

牽引の間，あなたの首（腰）を伸ばすために引く力が加わります．
During traction therapy, your neck [lower back] is given a pull in order to stretch the area.

`pull：引く力`

牽引は，椎間板の圧力を減らして痛みを抑える効果が望めます．
Traction reduces the intradiscal pressure and has pain-relieving effects.

牽引は，首の後ろ側の筋肉を伸ばします．
Traction stretches the muscles in the back of your neck.

症状と体重により安全な牽引の強さが定められています．
Safe strength of traction is defined according to the symptoms and the patient's body weight.

`be defined：定められる / according to～：～によって，～に従って`

これ以上強い牽引は危険です．
It is dangerous to give a stronger pull.

引っ張られる力は強すぎませんか．

Is it too strong?

強く引っ張ればいいというものではありません（より強く引っ張ればいい，と考える人たちがいますが，それは違います）．

Some people think a stronger pull is better, but it is not true.

途中でつらくなったらすぐに教えてください．

If you feel uneasy, please let me know immediately.

> uneasy：（体が）楽でない

≡ 温罨法，ホットパック

温罨法を行います．

Let's start the hot compress treatment.

> hot compress：温罨法

温罨法は患部を温めます．

Hot compress treatment warms up the injured area.

温罨法は，血行をよくして痛みを緩和する効果があります．

When a hot compress is applied, blood circulation improves and it has a pain-relieving effect.

温罨法をすると，患部が徐々にポカポカ温かくなり，血行をよくして痛みを和らげていきます．

When a hot compress is applied, you feel a comfortable level of warmth in the affected area. At the same time, your blood flow increases and the pain is relieved.

保湿することで電気療法が効率よく行えます（湿熱）．

After moisturizing the skin, electric therapy becomes more effective.

> moisturize：保湿する

熱かったり，何かあったりしたらすぐに言ってください．

If it is too hot, or if you feel something is wrong, please let me know immediately.

冷罨法，アイスパック

患部が炎症を起こしていますので，冷却します．/
患部の炎症を抑えるために，冷やします．
Since the injured area is inflamed, I will cool the area. /
In order to reduce the inflammation, I will cool the injured area.

寒冷療法（冷却）は，内出血を抑え，腫れや痛みを軽減する効果が望めます．
Cryotherapy reduces internal bleeding along with swelling and pain.

> cryotherapy：寒冷療法 / internal bleeding：内出血 / along with 〜：〜とともに

市販の湿布には冷却効果は望めません．
Commercially available plasters have no cooling effect. /
Non-prescription plasters have little cooling effect.

> commercially available：市販の / plaster：（貼るタイプの）湿布 / non-prescription：処方箋なしで購入可能な

冷やすと最初に痛く感じることが多いですが，1〜2分たつと痛みが薄らいできます．
Cooling often causes pain, but the pain eases after one or two minutes.

はじめは冷たく感じますが，徐々に慣れてきます．
It might feel very cold, but you will become used to it soon.

> be (become) used to 〜：〜に慣れる

冷たすぎませんか．
Is it too cold?

冷えすぎたらすぐに教えてください．
If it becomes too cold, please let me know.

冷たすぎたり，痛みを感じたりする場合はすぐに教えてください
If it is too cold, or if you feel pain, please let me know immediately.

痛みの感覚がなくなってきたら教えてください．
When you become insensitive to pain, please let me know.

> insensitive：無感覚な，感じない

マイクロ波療法を行います.
We will start the microwave therapy now.

`microwave therapy：マイクロ波療法`

マイクロ波は，患部の深部を刺激し，血流をよくします.
Microwaves stimulate the deeper part of the affected area and improve the blood flow.

マイクロ波治療は血流を改善し，治癒を促進します.
Microwave therapy improves the blood flow and promotes healing.

この治療は，服を着たままで受けられます*.
You can receive this treatment with your clothes on.

`with your clothes on：服を着たままで`
*ただし，ラメが入った服は燃えるので注意.

スマートフォンか携帯電話がポケットのなかに入っていませんか.
Do you have a smartphone or cellular phone in your pocket?

スマートフォンや携帯電話などの電子機器をマイクロは治療器に近づけないでください. それらの機器が壊れる場合があります.
Please do not place electronic devices, such as smartphones or cellular phones, near the microwave therapy equipment as they may get damaged.

`electronic device：電子機器`

湿布や金属製のアクセサリーは外してください. 熱傷が起きる可能性があります.
Please take off your plaster and metal accessories. They may cause a burn injury.

`burn injury：熱傷`

補聴器を外してください.
Please take off your hearing aid.

`take off：外す / hearing aid：補聴器`

運動療法の施術のための表現

Expressions for Exercise Therapy

Introduction

本章では，運動療法の効果の説明のための表現と，患者に身体を動かしてもらう時の表現を学びます．前者では，「運動療法は，低下した身体機能の回復に役立ちます．」（Exercise therapy helps restore decreased physical function.）のような表現が代表的な例です．後者では，「ゆっくりとこの筋肉を伸ばします．」（I will slowly stretch this muscle.）のような表現のヴァリエーションがあります．「もう少しです．頑張ってください．」（It is almost finished. You can do it.）のような励ましの表現も大事です．

運動療法の説明

これから運動療法を行います．
We will start the exercise therapy now.

運動療法は，低下した身体機能の回復に役立ちます．
Exercise therapy helps restore decreased physical function.

restore：回復する / decreased：低下した / physical function：身体機能

運動療法は，身体の運動機能の障害の除去を目的としています．
Exercise therapy aims to eliminate damage to the motor functions of the body.

aims to ～：～することをめざす / eliminate：なくす，除去する / motor function：運動機能

心疾患がある場合にはこの療法はお勧めできません．
If you have a heart condition or disease, this therapy is not recommended.

heart condition, heart disease：心臓病 / recommend：推薦する，勧める

運動療法は，体系的かつ計画された身体の動きを通して行われます．
Exercise therapy is performed through systematic and planned body movements.

運動療法には，全身運動療法と局所運動療法があります．

Exercise therapy includes whole-body exercise therapy and local exercise therapy.

whole-body exercise therapy：全身運動療法 / local exercise therapy：局所運動療法

全身運動療法は，全身の機能や体力の回復を図るものです．

Whole-body exercise therapy aims to restore the function and energy of the whole body.

全身運動療法は，局所障害の回復を間接的に促進します．

Whole-body exercise therapy indirectly promotes the recovery of local damage.

local damage：局所障害

局所運動療法は，筋力低下や関節可動域制限といった局所障害の回復を図ります．

Local exercise therapy aims to restore local damage, such as reduced muscle strength or a restricted range of joint motion.

restricted range of joint motion：関節可動域制限

運動療法の初期は，原則的に痛みを伴わない自動運動が推奨されます．

In the early stage of exercise therapy, in principle, painless active exercise is recommended.

painless：痛みのない

痛みを我慢して無理やり動かすと，骨化性筋炎を招きます．

If you put up with the pain and overexert your body, it will cause myositis ossificans.

myositis ossificans：骨化性筋炎

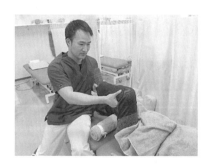

運動療法施術中の表現

痛みが出ない範囲で，可動域訓練や筋力トレーニングをします．

We will practice painless a range-of-motion exercise and do some muscle training.

range-of-motion exercise：可動域訓練

無理をしないでください．

Please do not push yourself. / Please do not overdo it.

push oneself：自分を追い込む

息苦しくなったら中止します．

If you get breathless, I will stop the therapy immediately.

get breathless：息苦しくなる

痛みを感じたら教えてください．

If you feel pain, please let me know.

自分の力だけで行ってください．

Please move your body by only using your own strength.

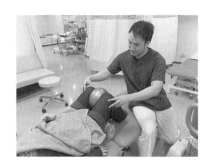

自分で動かさないでください．

Please do not move it by yourself.

抵抗に逆らって，押して（引いて）ください．

Please push [pull] against resistance.

resistance：抵抗

完全に力を抜いてください．

Please completely relax your whole body.

私がやってみせます．その後にご自身でもやってみましょう．

I will show you how to do it. Please do it by yourself.

息を止めないで行いましょう．

Please do it without holding your breath.

hold one's breath：息を止める

ゆっくりと数を数えながら行いましょう.
Let's do it, while counting slowly.

> count：数を数える

強かったら (つらかったら), (すぐに) 言ってください.
If it is too strong [hard] for you, please let me know (immediately).

もう少しです. 頑張ってください.
We are almost finished. / We will be done soon. You can do it.

≡ ストレッチング

ゆっくりとこの筋肉を伸ばします.
I will slowly stretch this muscle.

息を止めずにいてください.
Please do not hold your breath. / Please keep breathing.

深呼吸してください.
Please take a deep breath.

心地よく伸びていると感じたら言ってください.
When you feel that you can stretch your muscle comfortably, please let me know.

10 手技療法の施術のための表現

Expressions for Manipulation Therapy

本章では，手技療法の効果の説明のための表現と，患者の身体に触れて施術する時の表現を学びます．前者では，「手技療法は，さまざまな生体機能を活性化します．」（Manipulation therapy vitalizes the patient's various body functions.），「刺激が強ければいいというものではありません．」（Stronger stimulation is not necessarily good.）などの表現が代表的な例です．後者では，「筋肉が固くなっています．」（This muscle is stiff.）のような表現が必要になります．

手技療法の説明

手技療法は，徒手で施術する方法です．

Manipulation therapy is a method of treating an injury with one's bare hands.

> manipulation therapy：手技療法 / bare hand：徒手，素手

手技療法は，さまざまな生体機能を活性化します．

Manipulation therapy vitalizes the patient's various body functions.

> vitalize：活性化する / body function：生体機能

手技療法は，患者の自然治癒力を高めます．

Manipulation therapy improves the patient's natural healing powers.

> improve：改善する / natural healing power：自然治癒力

手技療法は，身体の自然治癒力を高めます．

Manipulation therapy activates the body's natural healing powers.

手技療法を通して，患者の身体機能が回復されます．

Through manipulation therapy, the patient's body functions are recovered.

> be recovered：回復される

手技療法は，傷ついた組織の回復を早めます．

Manipulation therapy quickens the recovery of injured cells.

quicken：早める，速める / recovery：回復 / injured cells：傷ついた細胞 → 傷ついた組織

手技療法は，損傷の早期回復を図るものです．

Manipulation therapy aims to facilitate the healing of injuries.

facilitate：促進する

多少の痛みを伴いますが，施術後は楽になります

It is slightly painful, but you will feel better after the treatment.

刺激が強ければいいというものではありません．

Stronger stimulation is not necessarily good.

not necessarily good：必ずしもよくはない

刺激が強ければ早く治るというわけではありません．

Some people think that stronger stimulation is better for the recovery of the injury, but it is not true.

some people think that 〜 , but it is not true：一部の人々は〜と考えますが，それは違います

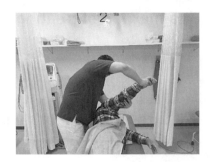

手技療法施術中の表現

刺激が強すぎるときは教えてください（刺激がきつかったら教えてください）．

When the stimulation is too strong, please let me know.

刺激が強すぎたり，弱すぎたりしたら，遠慮なく教えてください．

If the stimulation is too strong or too weak, please don't hesitate to let me know.

（強い）痛みが出たら教えてください.
If you feel (strong) pain, please let me know.

今押しているところに痛みはありますか.
Does it hurt when I press this point?

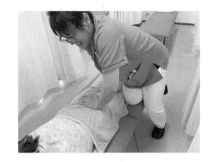

筋肉が固くなっています.
This muscle is stiff.

この姿勢がつらくなったら教えてください.
If it gets uneasy for you to keep this posture, please let me know.

posture：姿勢

処置・施術後の表現
Expressions for Post-Treatment Consultations

Introduction

処置・施術後の患者とのコミュケーションは，当日の処置・施術について患者の感想を聞き，今後の見通しと施術計画を説明し，日常生活での注意事項を伝えるものですから，とても大切です．「施術前より楽になっていますか．」(Are you feeling better than before the treatment?)，「継続して施術させてください．」(Please let me continue to treat you.)「患部を動かさないようにしてください．」(You must try not to move the injured part.) など，重要表現がたくさんあります．

施術直後・今後の見通し

施術前より楽になっていますか．/ 施術前と比べていかがですか．
Are you feeling better than before the treatment? /
How are you feeling now compared to before the treatment?

痛みが強くなっていませんか．
Hasn't the pain got more severe?

> more severe：よりひどい

→すぐに（そのうち，自然に）よくなりますか．
Will it go away soon [eventually / naturally]?

> eventually：そのうちに，結局は

→どれくらい長くかかりますか．
How long will it take to go away?

2～3日もすれば治ります．
It will go away in two or three days.

1週間くらいでより楽になるはずです．
You will probably feel better in about a week.

1〜2週間は大事をとったほうがいいです.
You have to be very careful for a week or two.

長くても10日くらいで自然に治るでしょう.
It will go away by itself within 10 days.

by itself：自動的に

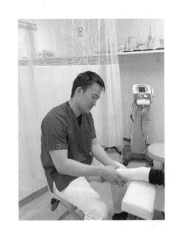

→それを聞いて, とても安心しました.
I'm relieved to hear that. / That's a relief.

relieved：安心する / relief：安堵, 安心

これは, 治るまでしばらくかかります.
It will take a while to go away.

take a while to 〜：〜するのにしばらく（時間が）かかる

これは加齢により引き起こされる患いです. ですから完全に治せません.
This is an affliction caused by aging. So it cannot be completely cured.

affliction：苦痛, 患い / aging：老化 / be cured：治癒される

☰ 指導管理

日常生活で痛む時があったら, 次の来院時に教えてください.
If you have pain in your daily life, please let me know during your next visit.

まだ症状が残っているので, 継続して施術させてください.
Since the symptom remains, we will have to continue the treatment.

since 〜：〜なので / remains：残っている

痛むようなら無理に動かさないほうがいいです.
If it hurts, it's better not to try to move it.

it's better not to 〜：〜しないほうがいい

今日一日はそっとしておいたほうがいいです.
It would be better not to do anything today.

しばらくの間，あまり無理をしないでください．

You shouldn't move it about too much for a while.

move 〜 about：〜をあちこちに動かす

たいしたことはありませんが，無理に首を動かさないようにしてください．

It doesn't seem to be serious, but you shouldn't move your neck too much.

膝のサポーターを着用したら，もっと快適に感じるかもしれません．

You might feel more comfortable if you wear a knee support.

support：サポーター

しばらく動かしてはいけません．

You mustn't move it for a while.

患部を動かさないようにしてください．

You must try not to move the injured part.

なるべく腕を上げておいてください．

Please keep your arm raised.

keep 〜 raised：〜を上げた状態にする

〈患者より〉
入浴してもいいですか．

May I take a bath?

→はい，いいですよ

Yes, you may take one.

one = bath

→今日はお風呂はやめておいてください．

Please refrain from taking a bath today.

refrain from 〜 ing：〜することを控える

冷湿布は役に立ちますか．

Does a cold plaster help?

→冷湿布も温湿布も患部を冷やしたり温めたりする効果があるわけではありません．

Both cold and warm plasters have no effect in cooling or warming the affected area.

→冷湿布も温湿布も鎮痛消炎効果をもつものです.

Both cold and warm plasters reduce pain and inflammation.

→冷湿布を貼ると,患部の皮膚が冷やされていると感じるのです.

If you apply a cold plaster, you feel that the skin in the affected area is cooled.

→明日からは患部を温めたほうが効果的です.

From tomorrow it would be better to keep the affected area warm.

→患部を冷やさないようにしたほうがいいです.

You should not cool the injured area.

cool：冷やす

→しばらくは,無理をしないで安静にしていたほうがいいです.

For a while, you shouldn't exert yourself and you should stay in bed.

exert oneself：無理をする

→もっとも快適な,何らかの姿勢で横になっていたほうがいいです.

You should lie down in whichever position feels most comfortable for you.

はい,そうします.

I'll do as you say.

入浴してマッサージするのはどうですか.

What about massaging it in the bath?

→入浴して温めるくらいなら構いません.

If you just take a bath and warm it up, it will be all right.

→軽い運動をすることを習慣づければ,痛みがいくらか和らぎます.

If you make it a habit to do light exercises, you will find the pain will somewhat alleviate.

make it a habit to ～：～することを習慣化する / light exercises：軽い運動 / you will find ～：～ということが分かるでしょう / alleviate：緩和する

どんな種類の運動ですか.
What kind of exercise?

→肩を運動させるべきです.
You should exercise [stretch] your shoulders.

→入浴する時に, 肩を動かすといいでしょう.
When you take a bath, you should move your shoulders about.

痛みのために寝られない時は, どうしたらいいでしょうか.
What should I do when I can't go to sleep because of the pain?

→わきの下に枕を置いたら, もっと楽になるでしょう.
You will feel more comfortable if you put a pillow under your armpits.

> **armpit：わきの下**

→寝る時は, 仰向けでなく, 膝を曲げて横向きで寝てみてください.
When you sleep, please do not lie on your back, but lie on your side with your legs bent.

> **with ～ bent：～を曲げられた状態で**

来月ゴルフに行くことにしていたのですが.
I was planning to play golf next month.

→スポーツはしばらく中止してください.
You will have to give up sports for a while.

> **give up：やめる, あきらめる**

残念ですが, 先生のおっしゃるとおりにします.
That's too bad, but I'll do as you say.

☰ 今後の通院に向けて

また, 明日見せに来てください.
Please visit us again tomorrow. / Please come again tomorrow. / Please come again to see us tomorrow.

また，明日患部の状態を見せに来てください.

Please let me assess the condition of the affected area tomorrow.

assess：診察する，評価する

明日は来られそうですか.

Can you come here [visit us] tomorrow?

何時ごろ来院できますか. / 何時頃なら来られそうですか.

What time can you come [visit us]?

次はいつ来られますか.

When can you come here [visit us] next time?

しばらく定期的に通えそうですか.

Can you visit [see] us on regular basis for the time being?

毎日通院してください.

I want you to come see us every day.

1日おきに通っていただけますか. / 当分の間，1日おきに通院してください.

**Can you come back to see us every other day? /
For the time being, you will have to visit here every other day.**

every other day：1日おきに

1週間おきに通院するようにしてください.

Be sure to come back to see us every other week.

来週また来てください.

Come again next week.

1週間後にまた来てください.

Please come back to see me a week from today.

a week from today：1週間後に

もしこの不具合が続くようであれば，また来てくだください.

If this trouble persists, come back again.

trouble：不具合 / persist：続く

なにか問題がありましたらご連絡ください.

Please let me know if there are any problems.

症状がよくならないようなら再来院してください.

Come and see me again if your condition doesn't improve.

come and see me：私に会いにきてください → 再来院してください

お大事にしてください（お大事にどうぞ）.

Please take care (of yourself).

すべて順調なら，もう通院の必要はありません.

If everything looks good, you won't have to come back again.

looks good：よく見える / won't = will not

処置・施術後の表現

会計のための表現

Expressions for Payment Procedures

Introduction

会計においては，「呼ばれたら受付で料金をお支払いください.」(When your name is called, please pay the fees at the reception desk.)のように, 接客英語の定型表現の多くが当てはまります. しかし,「初診の方なので, こちらの金額になります.」(This is your first visit, so it is this amount.),「月の最初の通院時には健康保険証を必ずお持ちください.」(Please be sure to bring your health insurance card at the first visit of each month.)のような医療関係ならではの表現は, 特別に覚えてください.

支払い

呼ばれたら受付で料金をお支払いください.

When your name is called, please pay the fees at the reception desk.

> fee：料金

こちらが本日の料金です.

The fee for today's visit is this.

> the fee for today's visit：本日の訪問に対する料金 → 本日の料金

本日の料金は, 1,825円です. / 合計1,825円です.

The fee for today's visit is 1,825 yen. / The total is 1,825 yen.

初診の方なので, こちらの金額になります.

This is your first visit, so it is this amount.

> amount：合計, 合計額

初診料金が加算されています

A first time visit charge has been added.

> first time visit charge：初診料金 / add：加える

お支払いは現金のみです．

Please pay by cash.

cash：現金

日本円でしかお支払いいただけません．

We only accept Japanese yen.

accept：受け入れる / yen：円

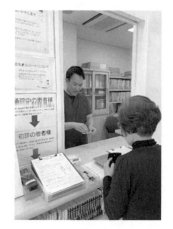

クレジットカードは使えますか．

Do you take credit cards?

クレジットカードはお使いになれません．

We don't accept credit cards.

今後の来院に向けて

次回の来院には，施術券を忘れずにお持ちください．

Please do not forget to bring your patient ID card to your next visit.

bring：持ってくる / next visit：次回の来院

施術券に電話番号が書いてあります．緊急の際にはご連絡ください．

Our telephone number is printed on your patient ID card. Please contact us in case of an emergency.

月の最初の通院時には健康保険証を必ずお持ちください．

Please be sure to bring your health insurance card at the first visit of each month.

be sure to ～：必ず～してください

あいさつ

お大事にしてください．

See you. / Take care. / Please take care. / Please take good care of yourself.

付　録

付録（1）：身体部位の英語名

頭部

髪	hair
額	forehead
頭	head
後頭部	back of the head
顔	face
首	neck
首筋, うなじ	nape
喉	throat
目	eye
耳	ear
頬	cheek
顎関節	jaw
鼻	nose
口	mouth
顎先	chin

体幹（trunk）

肩	shoulder
肩甲帯	shoulder girdle
腋窩, わき	armpit
胸部	chest
乳房	breast
腹部	abdomen
へそ	navel
ウエスト	waist
背中	back
腰	hip / lower back
殿部	buttock

上肢（upper limb）

上腕	upper arm
肘	elbow
前腕	forearm
手首	wrist
手	hand
指	finger
親指	thumb
人差し指	forefinger
中指	middle finger
薬指	ring finger
小指	little finger

下肢（lower limb）

脚	leg
大腿	thigh
下腿	crus
膝	knee
脛	shin
ふくらはぎ	calf
足首	ankle
足	foot
甲	instep
踵	heel
足の裏	sole
土踏まず	arch of the foot
足の親指	big toe

左ページに提示された英語のなかに，知らなかった単語や忘れていた単語があれば，
下のイラストの該当箇所に書き込んでください.

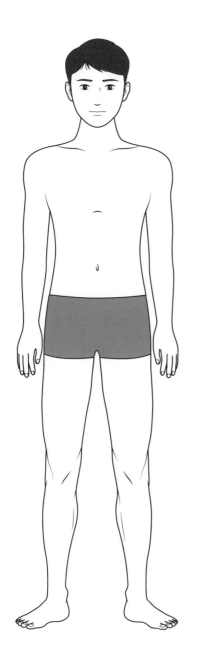
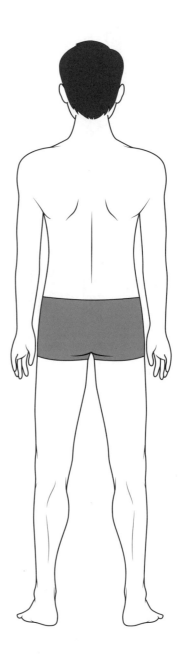

付録（2）：筋肉の英語名

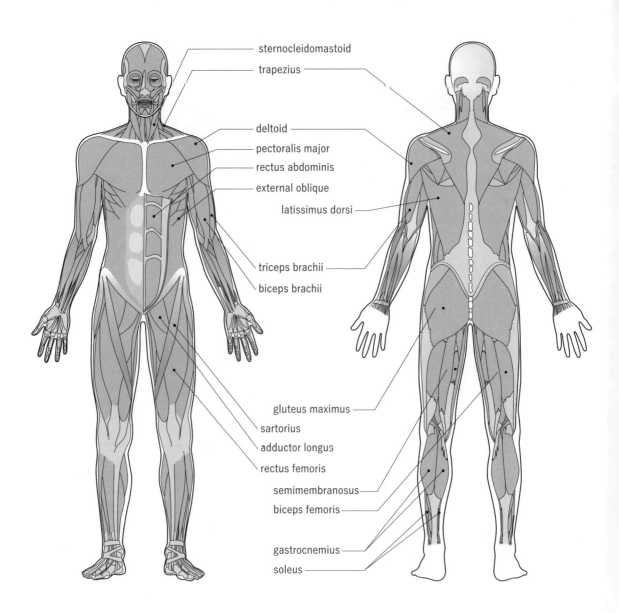

sternocleidomastoid

trapezius

deltoid

pectoralis major

rectus abdominis

external oblique

latissimus dorsi

triceps brachii

biceps brachii

gluteus maximus

sartorius

adductor longus

rectus femoris

semimembranosus

biceps femoris

gastrocnemius

soleus

頭部

側頭筋	temporal
眼輪筋	orbicularis oculi
咬筋	masseter
口輪筋	orbicularis oris
笑筋	risorius
胸鎖乳突筋	sternocleidomastoid

肩関節周囲

三角筋	deltoid
烏口腕筋	coracobrachialis
肩甲下筋	subscapularis
棘上筋	supraspinatus
棘下筋	infraspinatus
大円筋	teres major
小円筋	teres minor
肩甲挙筋	levator scapulae
僧帽筋	trapezius
大菱形筋	rhomboid major
小菱形筋	rhomboid minor
広背筋	latissimus dorsi
中殿筋	gluteus medius

上肢帯

鎖骨下筋	subclavius
前鋸筋	serratus anterior
大胸筋	pectoralis major
小胸筋	pectoralis minor
腹直筋	rectus abdominis
外腹斜筋	external oblique

肘関節周囲

上腕筋	brachii
上腕二頭筋	biceps brachii
上腕三頭筋	triceps brachii
肘筋	anconeus
腕橈骨筋	brachioradialis
長掌筋	palmaris longus
円回内筋	pronator teres
回外筋	supinator
長母指屈筋	flexor pollicis longus (finger flexors)
長母指伸筋	extensor pollicis longus (finger extensors)
長母指外転筋	abductor pollicis longus
方形回内筋	pronator quadratus

下肢帯

縫工筋	sartorius
長内転筋	adductor longus
大腿直筋	rectus femoris
外側広筋	vastus lateralis
内側広筋	vastus medialis
前脛骨筋	tibialis anterior
大殿筋	gluteus maximus
半膜様筋	semimembranosus
大腿二頭筋	biceps femoris
大内転筋	adductor magnus
薄筋	gracilis
腓腹筋	gastrocnemius
ヒラメ筋	soleus
アキレス腱	Achilles tendon

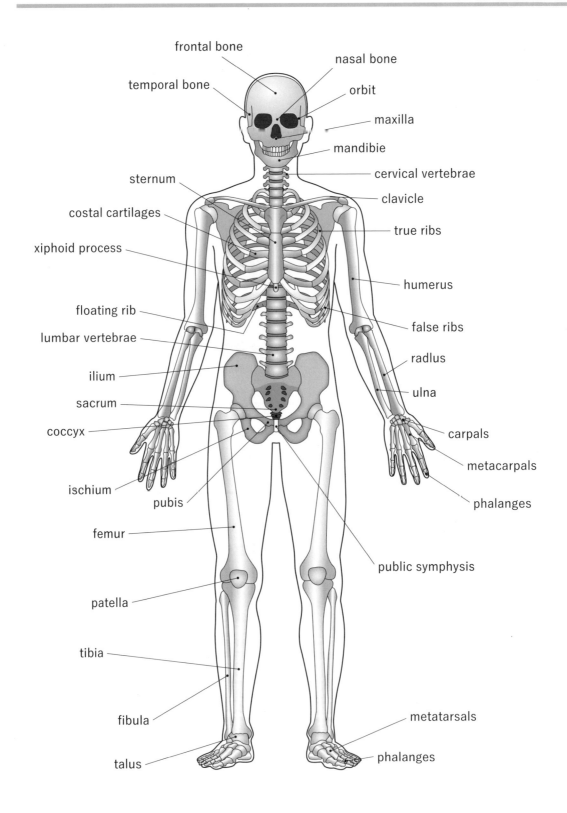

frontal bone

nasal bone

temporal bone

orbit

maxilla

mandibie

cervical vertebrae

sternum

clavicle

costal cartilages

true ribs

xiphoid process

humerus

floating rib

false ribs

lumbar vertebrae

radlus

ilium

ulna

sacrum

coccyx

carpals

ischium

metacarpals

pubis

phalanges

femur

public symphysis

patella

tibia

fibula

metatarsals

talus

phalanges

頭部

頭蓋骨	skull / cranium
頭頂骨	parietal bone
前頭骨	frontal bone
側頭骨	temporal bone
後頭骨	occipital bone
上顎骨	maxilla
下顎骨	mandible
鼻骨	nasal bone
蝶形骨	sphenoid
頬骨	zygomatic bone
眼窩	orbit

上肢帯

頸椎	cervical vertebrae
鎖骨	clavicle
胸骨	sternum
肋軟骨	costal cartilage
剣状突起	xiphoid process
肩甲骨	scapula
胸椎	thoracic vertebrae
腰椎	lumbar vertebrae
肋骨	ribs
真性肋骨	true rib
浮遊肋骨	floating rib
仮肋	false rib

肘関節周囲

上腕骨	humerus
橈骨	radius
尺骨	ulna
手根骨	carpal
中手骨	metacarpal
指骨	phalange

骨盤周囲

骨盤	pelvis
腸骨	ilium
坐骨	ischium
恥骨	pubis / pubic bone
恥骨結合	public symphysis
仙骨	sacrum
尾骨	coccyx

下肢帯

大腿骨	femur
膝蓋骨	patella
脛骨	tibia
腓骨	fibula
距骨	talus
踵骨	calcaneus
足根骨	tarsal bones
中足骨	metatarsal

Medical Questionnaire　事前質問票

	Reception Date 受付日		Year 年	Month 月	Day 日

Name 氏名	Family Name	First Name	Sex 性別	☐　Male　男 ☐　Female　女
Date of Birth 生年月日	Year 年　　Month 月　　Day 日		Age 年齢	Years old 歳
Nationality　国籍		Language　言語		

Where in your body do you have symptoms?　症状があるのはどの部位ですか.

Please circle the affected area(s) in the diagram below.　症状のある部位に○をしてください.

When did you first notice the symptoms?　その症状には最初にいつ気がつきましたか.

Approximately だいたい	Year 年	Month 月	Day 日	☐　Morning 午前	☐　Afternoon 午後

Where did it happen?　それはどこで起きましたか.

☐　Home　自宅　　　　　☐　Workplace　職場　　　　☐　School　学校
☐　Street　道路　　　　　☐　I don't know.　分からない
☐　Other　その他　　　　[　　　　　　　　　　　　　　　　　　　　　　　　　　　　　]

What were you doing when you got injured?　受傷した時なにをしていましたか.

☐　Walking　歩いていた　　☐　Running　走っていた　　☐　Standing立っていた
☐　Sitting　座っていた　　☐　Lying down　横になっていた
☐　Going up or down the stairs　階段を上り下りしていた　☐　Working　仕事中
☐　Doing sports　スポーツをしていた　　　　　　　　　☐　I don't know.　分からない
☐　Other　その他　　　　[　　　　　　　　　　　　　　　　　　　　　　　　　　　　　]

How did the injury occur?　どのようにしてけがをしたのですか（痛めましたか）.

☐　Fell to the ground　転んだ　　☐　Stumbled　つまずいた　　☐　Slipped　滑った
☐　Bumped into something or someone　～にぶつかった　　☐　Misstepped　踏み外した
☐　Fell down on my hands or knee　手や膝をついた　　☐　Twisted　捻った
☐　Jammed my finger　指をついた　　　　　　　　　　☐　I don't know.　分からない
☐　Other　その他　　　［　　　　　　　　　　　　　　　　　　　　　　　　　　］

What kind of symptoms do you have?　どんな症状がありますか.

☐　Pain　痛み　　☐　Bruise　打撲　　☐　Swelling　腫れ　　☐　Fever　熱
☐　Numbness　しびれ　　　　　☐　Dislocation　脱臼　　☐　Nausea　吐き気
☐　I don't know.　分からない　　☐　Other　その他　　　［　　　　　　　　　　］

What kind of pain do you have?　どんな痛みがありますか.

☐　Throbbing pain　ズキンズキンという痛み　　☐　Stabbing pain　刺すような痛み
☐　Burning pain　焼けるような痛み　　　　　　☐　Shooting pain　痛みが走る
☐　Continued pain　持続する痛み　　　　　　　☐　I don't know.　分からない
☐　Other　その他　　　［　　　　　　　　　　　　　　　　　　　　　　　　　　］

How severe is the pain?　痛みの強さはどれくらいですか.

Tolerable　←　0　1　2　3　4　5　6　7　8　9　10　→　Intolerable
我慢できる　　　　　　　　　　　　　　　　　　　　　　　　　　　我慢できない

When do the symptoms occur?　どんな時に症状が出ますか.

☐　Morning　朝　　☐　Noon　昼　　☐　Evening　夕方　　☐　Night　夜
☐　Irregularly　不定期に　　☐　Suddenly　突然に　　☐　Constantly　いつも
☐　When moving the affected area　患部を動かす時　　☐　When pushed　押された時
☐　When resting　安静にしている時　　☐　When lying down　横になっている時
☐　When walking　歩いている時　　　　☐　When waking up　起床時
☐　I don't know.　分からない　☐　Other　その他　　　［　　　　　　　　　　　　］

Check the appropriate boxes below.　当てはまるところにチェックしてください.

☐　Pacemaker　ペースメーカー　　　　　　☐　Artificial joint　人工関節
☐　Stent　ステント
☐　High blood pressure　高血圧　　　　　☐　Low blood pressure　低血圧
☐　Allergy to cotton　綿アレルギー　　　　☐　Allergy to nylon　ナイロンアレルギー
☐　Allergy to adhesive tape　粘着テープアレルギー
☐　Pregnant　妊娠中　　☐　Other　その他　　　［　　　　　　　　　　　　　　］

Are you taking any medication?　何かお薬を飲んでいますか.

☐　No.　いいえ　☐　Yes.　はい　　　［　　　　　　　　　　　　　　　　　　　］

（本文 p9）

付録（5）：登録用紙（施術申込書）

Patient Registration Form 登録用紙（施術申込書）

			Reception Date 受付日		Year 年		Month 月	Day 日

Name 氏名	Family Name First Name		Sex 性別	☐ Male 男 ☐ Female 女
Date of Birth 生年月日	Year 年	Month 月	Day 日	Age 年齢	Years old 歳

Address or Accommodation in Japan   日本での滞在先

Address in Home Country〈For Short-term Visitors Only〉   母国での住所〈短期滞在者のみ〉

Phone No. 電話番号	Home 家	Occupation 職業
	Mobile 携帯	

Nationality 国籍	Native Language 母語

Languages You Speak 対応できる言語

Emergency Contact Details 緊急連絡先	
Name 氏名	Relationship 患者との関係
Address 住所	
Phone No. 電話番号	Home 家	Mobile 携帯

Immigration Status in Japan 日本での滞在状況		
☐ Resident 居住 ☐ Vacation 旅行 ☐ Other その他	☐ Short Stay 短期滞在 ☐ Student 学生	☐ Business 仕事

Type of Health Insurance   保険の種類

☐ Japanese Health Insurance 日本の保険   ☐ Public 公的保険   ☐ Private 民間保険
☐ Overseas Health Insurance 海外の保険
　　Name of Insurance Company 保険会社名

☐ Uninsured 保険に加入していない
* Please present your health insurance card or elated documents if available.
　保険証か関連書類をお持ちでしたらご提示ください.

（本文 p6）

用語一覧

深呼吸する：take a deep breath

【著者略歴】

塩　川　春　彦
（しお　かわ　はる　ひこ）

1996年　信州大学大学院教育学研究科修了
1999年　北海学園大学経済学部助教授
2000年　北海学園大学経済学部教授
2003年　北海学園大学経営学部教授
2010年　帝京科学大学医療科学部教授
2019年　帝京科学大学教育人間学部教授（〜2021年）

【監修者略歴】

杉　山　　渉
（すぎ　やま　わたる）

1976年　日本大学歯学部卒業
1980年　日本大学大学院歯学研究科修了
2011年　日本大学歯学部兼任講師（〜現在）
2014年　帝京科学大学医療科学部教授
　　　　歯科医師，柔道整復師，柔道整復師専科教員，柔道整復実技審査員，認定柔道整復師

小　黒　正　幸
（お　ぐろ　まさ　ゆき）

1994年　二松学舎大学国際政治経済学部卒業
2011年　帝京千住接骨院院長
2012年　帝京科学大学医療科学部非常勤講師
2016年　帝京科学大学医療科学部助教
2019年　人間総合科学大学大学院人間総合科学研究科修了
2022年　帝京科学大学医療科学部講師
　　　　柔道整復師，柔道整復師専科教員，柔道整復実技審査員

柔道整復師のための英会話表現　　ISBN 978-4-263-24093-9

2022年10月25日　第1版第1刷発行

執筆代表　塩　川　春　彦
監　　修　杉　山　　渉
　　　　　小　黒　正　幸
発行者　　白　石　泰　夫
発行所　　医歯薬出版株式会社
〒113-8612　東京都文京区本駒込1-7-10
TEL.（03）5395-7641（編集）・7616（販売）
FAX.（03）5395-7624（編集）・8563（販売）
https://www.ishiyaku.co.jp/
郵便振替番号 00190-5-13816

乱丁・落丁の際はお取り替えいたします　　印刷・壮光舎印刷／製本・愛千製本所